Critical Issues in Family Practice

Kenneth P. Kushner received his B.A. from the University of Wisconsin and his M.A. and Ph.D. in Clinical Psychology from the University of Michigan. From 1977 to 1981 he was an assistant professor in the departments of Family Medicine and Psychiatry at the Medical College of Ohio. In 1981, Dr. Kushner served as a lecturer for the University of Maryland's Far East Division in Yokosuka, Japan. He is currently a clinical assistant professor in the Department of Family Medicine and Practice at the University of Wisconsin Medical School and is on the staff of the Wisconsin Family Studies Institute. In addition, he retains an appointment as a clinical assistant professor at the Medical College of Ohio. Dr. Kushner was president of the Society of Psychologists in Family Practice and Primary Health Care from 1979–1981.

Harry E. Mayhew graduated from the University of Michigan Medical School and practiced family medicine in St. Clair, Michigan for fifteen years. After serving as assistant director of the E. W. Sparrow Hospital Family Practice Residency in Lansing, Michigan, and assistant professor at the College of Human Medicine at Michigan State University, he became professor and chairman of the Department of Family Medicine at Medical College of Ohio in 1976. Under his direction, the department developed and maintains an active undergraduate program, a medical college family practice residency, and four affiliated community hospital family practice residency programs. Dr. Mayhew is a Diplomate of the American Board of Family Practice, a Fellow of the American Academy of Family Physicians, and a consultant for the Residency Assistance Program.

Leroy A. Rodgers holds a B.S. in psychology and pre-medical studies from Allegheny College and an M.D. from Temple University Health Sciences Center. Following internship, he practiced general and family medicine for seven years as chairman of Family Practice Associates in Portage, Pennsylvania. From 1974 to 1977, Dr. Rodgers was Director of Ambulatory Care and Community Medicine at Conemaugh Valley Memorial Hospital, Johnstown, Pennsylvania. He accepted his present position as associate professor and vice chairman of the Department of Family Medicine at the Medical College of Ohio in September, 1977. He currently also serves as Chief of Staff at the Medical College of Ohio Hospital, Executive Medical Director of the Northwest Ohio Developmental Center, and Medical Director of the Lucas County Corrections Center. Dr. Rodgers is a past president of the Pennsylvania Academy of Family Physicians, a Diplomate of the American Board of Family Practice, and a Fellow of the American Academy of Family Physicians.

Rita L. Hermann graduated from Columbia University School of Social Work in 1969. She then was employed as a clinical social worker for the Huron Valley Child Guidance Clinic of the Washtenaw County Community Mental Health Center in Ann Arbor, Michigan and later as the supervisor of children's services in one of the three catchment programs of the Mental Health Center. Ms. Hermann joined the faculty of the Medical College of Ohio in 1978 as an assistant professor. She has assisted in the behavioral science training of residents and medical students as well as performing clinical services. Ms. Hermann is a member of the National Association of Social Workers, the Academy of Certified Social Workers, and the Society of Teachers of Family Medicine.

Critical Issues in Family Practice

Cases and Commentaries

Editors

Kenneth P. Kushner, Ph.D.
Harry E. Mayhew, M.D.
Leroy A. Rodgers, M.D.
Rita L. Hermann, M.S.S.W.

Foreword by G. Gayle Stephens, M.D.

Springer Publishing Company
New York

Springer Publishing Company, Inc.
200 Park Avenue South
New York, New York 10003

82 83 84 85 86 / 10 9 8 7 6 5 4 3 2 1

Library of Congress Cataloging in Publication Data
Main entry under title:

Critical issues in family practice.

    Includes bibliographies and index.
    1. Family medicine—Case studies.   2. Family medicine—Psychological aspects—Case studies.   3. Physician and patient—Case studies.   4. Interpersonal relations—Case studies.   I. Kushner, Kenneth P.   [DNLM: 1. Family practice.   WB 110 C934]
R729.5.G4C74   1982   616'.09   82-5943
ISBN 0-8261-3660-5   AACR2
ISBN 0-8261-3661-3 (pbk.)

Printed in the United States of America

Contents

Section IV: The Practice

Foreword

A book like this one is long overdue in Family Practice. It is much nearer the "state of the art" in our field than attempted compendia, encyclopedic tomes that are but pale copies of textbooks of medicine, or treatises on the politics, economics or philosophy of family medicine.

This is essentially a book of stories, real-life stories about the clinical experiences of family physicians: patient care, relationships with consultants, relationships between residents and supervisors and peers, and relationships with nurses and other co-professionals. Each is interesting, relevant, and rich in lessons about enduring issues that can never be learned too well.

The format is deceptively simple. A story is told in first person by a resident, faculty or practitioner, about his/her experience with a particular patient, consultant or colleague. Each has the unmistakable ring of truth, readily recognizable by any physician, who inevitably will be reminded of his/her own stories. These accounts are fresh and candid, courageously exposing what is usually unspeakable—failures, ignorance, impulsivity, naivete, anger, guilt, narcissism, and other human foibles and idiosyncrasies. There is no attempt to hide or evade what happened.

Each account is followed by commentaries from two reactors, who have nothing to go on except the story as given. Each commentator analyzes the dilemmas, problems and impasses in a very personal way, while also bringing to bear information from the literature.

The acquisition of these 34 anecdotes is a major achievement, requiring three years of solicitation, editing and organizing. This tells us that the task was not simple, but in these accounts the editors have accrued an enormous amount of grist to be ground into meal.

One can imagine a dozen uses for this material in teaching and practice. The timeless character of the "critical incidents" makes them profound and superficial, complex and simple; all instructive. The editors have tampered with their material as little as possible. This makes for unevenness of style and projects a broad range of literary skill, but it preserves the vitality and realism of the true experiences.

From such stories, and our attempts to understand them, comes the foundation in reality upon which the superstructure of our discipline can be erected. Deceptively simple, but also deceptively profound. Every discipline in medicine has its own unique stories, paradigms and prototypes, that ultimately come to constitute the stuff of the discipline. By-passing this stage of development would be fatal.

It is a personal pleasure for me to have been allowed to read this book in manuscript form and write this foreword. These editors are on the right trail. I hope that their book will be disseminated widely and that they will follow through on their promise of another volume. When we have learnt these stories by heart, and have no more need for them, the discipline of Family Practice will have passed the test of distinctiveness, and we will need no longer to hear the plaintive question, nor feel the sting of incredulous skepticism.

G. Gayle Stephens, M.D.

Contributors

To provide anonymity, the contributors of incidents are listed below in alphabetical order. Their names are not given with the incidents they contributed.

Andreas S. Ahbel, M.D., Private Family Practice, Canton, Ohio

Joseph Baum, M.D., Private Family Practice, Manchester, Iowa

Ross R. Black, II, M.D., Associate Director, Family Practice Center, Akron City Hospital, Akron, Ohio

Zorena S. Bolton, M.S.S.W., Coordinator, Behavioral Science Program, Family Practice Residency, Central Texas Medical Foundation, Austin, Texas

Howard Brody, M.D., Ph.D., Assistant Professor, Family Practice and Philosophy, and Assistant Coordinator, Medical Humanities Program, Michigan State University, East Lansing, Michigan

Michael L. Coates, M.D., Assistant Professor of Family Medicine, University of Virginia School of Medicine, Charlottesville, Virginia

Jonathan Cree, MRCGP, M.A., Adjunct Associate Professor of Family Medicine, UCLA Family Practice Residency Program, Antelope Valley Medical Center, Lancaster, California

William G. Fenner, M.D., Assistant Director, Family Practice Residency Program, Bon Secours Hospital, Grosse Point, Michigan

James A. Ferrante, M.D., Director, Family Practice Residency Program, St. Margaret Memorial Hospital, Pittsburgh, Pennsylvania

Carl Flaxer, M.D., Private Family Practice, Commerce City, Colorado

John C. Gillen, M.D., Professor and Chairman, Department of Family Practice, Wright State University School of Medicine, Dayton, Ohio

Robert D. Gillette, M.D., Associate Professor, Department of Family Medicine, University of Cincinnati, Cincinnatti, Ohio

Glen R. Johnson, M.D., Director, Family Practice Residency, Central Texas Medical Foundation, Austin, Texas

Brian L. Jones, M.B., Ch.B., FRCGP (NZ), Director of Residency Training, Section of Family Medicine, Brown University, The Memorial Hospital, Pawtucket, Rhode Island

Harry E. Mayhew, M.D., Professor and Chairman, Department of Family Medicine, Medical College of Ohio, Toledo, Ohio

Henry R. Silverman, Jr., M.D., Private Family Practice, Associate Clinical Professor, Department of Family Medicine, Medical College of Ohio, Toledo, Ohio

Mary C. Spaulding, M.D., Navajo Nation Health Foundation, Sage Memorial Hospital, Ganado, Arizona

Jon K. Sternburg, M.D., Clinical Assistant Professor, Temple University, Highland Physicians, Ltd., Honesdale, Pennsylvania

Robert B. Taylor, M.D., Associate Professor, Department of Family and Community Medicine, Bowman Gray School of Medicine, Winston-Salem, North Carolina

Thomas U. Todd, M.D., Private Family Practice, Cincinnati, Ohio

Robert L. Urata, M.D., Community Clinic, National Health Services Corps, Seattle, Washington

James P. Villotti, M.D., Private Family Practice, Englewood, Florida, Former Chief Family Practice Resident, Medical College of Ohio, Toledo, Ohio

Samuel W. Warburton, M.D., Associate Professor, Department of Community and Family Medicine, Duke University Medical Center, Durham, North Carolina

Charles H. Wile, M.D., Assistant Program Director, USAF Family Practice Training Program, Eglin Air Force Base, Eglin, Florida

Thaddeus Zdanowicz, M.D., Private Practice, Shumpert Medical Center, Shreveport, Louisiana, and Former Chief Family Practice Resident, Medical College of Ohio, Toledo, Ohio

Charles R. Zimont, M.D., Private Family Practice, Constantine, Michigan

Commentators

The names of the authors of the commentaries on the incidents contained in this book are listed below. The name, title, and affiliation of each commentator are cited at the end of his/her respective commentary.

Michael J. Asken, Ph.D.
Richard M. Baker, M.D.
B. Lewis Barnett, Jr., M.D.
Ronald E. Benson, Ph.D.
Ross R. Black, II, M.D.
Howard Brody, M.D., Ph.D.
Elsa L. Brown, R.N., Ph.D.
Paul C. Brucker, B.S., M.D.
Allan H. Bruckheim, M.D.
Philip Caravella, M.D.
Grace H. Chickadonz, R.N., Ph.D.
John H. Coleman, M.D.
Hiram Benjamin Curry, M.D.
George Darah, D.O.
Don E. DeWitt, M.D.
John L. Duhring, M.D.
Alan L. Evans, Ph.D.
Charles E. Fenlon, M.D.
James A. Ferrante, M.D.
Lane A. Gerber, Ph.D.
John P. Geyman, M.D.
Marvin E. Gottlieb, M.D.
Richard I. Haddy, M.D.
Rita L. Hermann, M.S.S.W.
Joseph W. Hess, M.D.
David L. Hoff, M.D.
David M. Holden, M.D.
B. Leslie Huffman, Jr., M.D.
Larry W. Johnson, M.D.
Roland T. Keddie, M.D., J.D.
John P. Kemph, M.D.

Timothy D. Krugh, J.D.
Kenneth P. Kushner, Ph.D.
David N. Little, M.D.
Hugh James Lurie, M.D.
Denis J. Lynch, Ph.D.
Chris D. Marquart, M.D.
Harry E. Mayhew, M.D.
Jack H. Medalie, M.D., M.P.H.
Joel H. Merenstein, M.D.
William T. Merkel, Ph.D.
J. David Michaels, B.S., PA-C
Charles E. Morrill, M.D.
Lewis B. Morrow, M.D.
Henry C. Mullins, M.D.
Sam A. Nixon, M.D.
Daniel J. Ostergaard, M.D.
Warren H. Pearse, M.D.
Lynn A. Phelps, M.D.
James G. Price, M.D.
Jorge Prieto, M.D.
Gary E. Ruoff, M.D.
D. Henry Ruth, M.D.
Brian Schmitt, M.D.
Erica R. Serlin, Ph.D.
Joy D. Skeel, B.S. Nsg., M. Div.
Frank F. Snyder, M.D.
G. Gayle Stephens, M.D.
Robert B. Taylor, M.D.
Neil R. Thomford, M.D.
Clinton H. Toewe, II, M.D.
Donna Ailport Woodson, M.D.
Joel P. Zrull, M.D.

Introduction

The concept and development of this book paralleled the growth of the Department of Family Medicine at the Medical College of Ohio. In 1976, Harry E. Mayhew, M.D. became the first full-time chairman and was soon joined by the three other editors: Kenneth P. Kushner, Ph.D.; Leroy A. Rodgers, M.D.; and Rita L. Hermann, M.S.S.W. One of the major tasks of the new faculty was to establish curricula for residency education. Like all family practice residencies, an active behavioral science program was established.

Before any residents were accepted, we began to define what in the very broad field of behavioral science we wanted to teach and how we intended to teach it. We were impressed by the work of Balint (1972) and agreed that behavioral science would be best taught in reference to current cases of the residents and faculty.

As we began to discuss our own and the residents' cases, we noticed a very intriguing phenomenon. Certain cases stood out because of the affective impact that they had upon the physician. Typically, this impact originated in situations with psychosocial dimensions that created strong emotions, such as frustration, uncertainty, anxiety, or anger. For lack of another term, we began to call the situations which provoked such psychosocial dilemmas "critical incidents."

We continued to notice an increasing educational value in the concept of the critical incident. When a resident presented a case which provoked a strong emotional component, he or she was motivated to learn about the psychosocial issues involved in the case. The high degree of uncertainty created by the critical incident provided a "teachable moment." With the help of Dr. Ronald Benson, an ethicist who spent a sabbatical leave in the department, we experimented with a standardized form in which physicians re-corded situations they deemed to be critical incidents. We then discussed these incidents with the residents in a seminar similar to the Balint style. The discussions of these cases frequently provided the structure of our behavioral science seminars.

As we discussed our observations regarding critical incidents with experi-enced physicians, we noticed another interesting phenomenon. Many physi-cians were interested in describing similar types of incidents that they them-selves had experienced during their careers. Even though events they related occurred many years earlier, they still seemed very much alive in the minds of the physicians, due, in large part, to the fact that the incident and the issues it had raised remained incompletely or unsatisfactorily resolved. Often the physicians seemed to relive the emotions which were evoked in the original incident. We began to see considerable merit in finding a forum in which experienced physicians could discuss their critical incidents with physicians in training. We thought that this would provide a way of teaching the art of medicine as seen through the eyes of the experienced family physician.

We examined primary care literature to see if there were precedents in this approach to teaching behavioral science. At the time, numerous books on psychiatry and/or behavioral science for the primary care physician were being published. While there is considerable value in many of these books, they lacked the specificity and the immediacy that we felt would be provided by a case book of critical incidents. We also found case books of ethical issues in medicine. However, our concept of critical incidents included more than just ethical dilemmas. In addition, most of these books seemed geared more toward the secondary or tertiary care specialist than to the family physician.

The work of Corsini and his associates came to our attention (Bermosk & Corsini, 1973; Calia & Corsini, 1972; Corsini & Howard, 1964; and Standal & Corsini, 1959). They had published a series of case books of critical incidents in other professions: nursing, school counseling, teaching and psychotherapy. Reviewing these books made us aware of the value and feasibility of writing a case book of critical incidents in family medicine. Our indebtedness to Corsini and his associates in terms of inspiration and methodology is gratefully ac-knowledged.

In the summer of 1978, three surveys were sent out, in which we asked practicing family physicians to send us descriptions of situations that they considered to be "critical incidents." The first mailing was to a group of 227 physicians who were acquaintances the authors thought might be interested in participating. The second mailing was to 452 members of the Ohio Academy of Family Physicians who reside in Northwest Ohio. The third mailing was sent to the directors of the 457 family practice residencies in the United States and Canada. The directors were asked to share our request for participation with their residents and faculty. At no time did we consider our sampling procedures to be scientific in nature. Rather, from the outset we had viewed this as largely being a convenience sample.

By July of 1979, a total of 68 descriptions of critical incidents had been received. While we were disappointed with the number of responses, we were extremely pleased with the quality of the incidents that we had received. Specific recruiting was done to obtain the incidents involving malpractice and nonpayment. From the original 68 incidents, we selected a subsample of 34 incidents that we thought would make an interesting, representative, and diverse collection for this book.

After finalizing the collection of incidents, we began the process of recruiting commentators. In each case people were chosen who either had national reputations, special expertise, and/or interest in the issues raised by the incident. For most incidents, two commentators were chosen, with at least one being a family physician. The commentators were sent copies of the incident with a model commentary, and were asked to critically examine the incident. In some instances the incidents were edited before they were sent to the commentators. In such cases, we endeavored to limit our editorial changes to grammatical corrections so as not to interfere with the meaning intended by the author of the incident. In preparing the final manuscript for publication, we found that we also had to make simple editorial changes in commentaries. Again, we tried to limit such changes.

One editorial policy that was difficult for us and which deserves special mention concerns the use of masculine pronouns. Our original intention was to edit the manuscript so that neutral expressions of gender such as he/she would be used, when appropriate, in place of their masculine counterparts. However, this often resulted in awkward sentence constructions. For that reason we have generally kept the masculine pronouns for the sake of clarity and style.

This volume of 34 incidents and their commentaries is the culmination of three years of work. Over this period of time we have received assistance without which we could not have completed the project. We would like to express our gratitude to the following people: Dorothy Woodward for her dedicated clerical assistance and manuscript preparation; Carol Hardt, Shirley Irving, Elizabeth Henderson, and Jane Kuns for secretarial help; B. Leslie Huffman, M.D., who wrote the letter that was sent in our mailing to the physicians of Northwest Ohio; the Medical College of Ohio and the Department of Family Medicine, which provided invaluable support; those who served as commentators in this book; and last but not least, those who shared their critical incidents.

This book does not mark the end of our study of critical incidents in family medicine. Rather, we view it as the first step. Since completing this manu-

script, we have received additional critical incidents. In addition, we anticipate that our readers might find that they have encountered or will encounter
critical incidents that they would like to share with other physicians. For that
reason, we would like to write a second volume of *Critical Issues in Family
Practice: Cases and Commentaries*. We invite our readers to contribute
incidents for it. For those who are interested, instructions for the submission
of critical incidents are on page xviii.

The Editors

References

Balint, M. *The doctor, his patient, and the illness*. New York: International
   Universities Press, 1972.
Bermosk, L. S., & Corsini, R. J. *Critical incidents in nursing*. Philadelphia:
   Saunders, 1973.
Calia, V. F., & Corsini, R. J. *Critical incidents in school counseling*. Engle-
   wood Cliffs, New Jersey: Prentice-Hall, 1972.
Corsini, R. J., & Howard, D. D. *Critical incidents in teaching*. Englewood
   Cliffs, New Jersey: Prentice-Hall, 1964.
Standal, S. W., & Corsini, R. J. *Critical incidents in psychotherapy*. Engle-
   wood Cliffs, New Jersey: Prentice-Hall, 1959.

How to Use This Book

The purpose of this book is to stimulate critical and creative thinking on the management of difficult situations that confront physicians. In order to get the most out of this book we recommend that you first read an incident and then, before reading the commentaries, ask yourself the following questions: How would I have felt if I had been in the same situation? What would I have done differently? What advice or suggestions would I give to the author of the incident? Can I think of similar situations that I, or my colleagues, have encountered? After you have answered these questions, read the commentaries. Do you agree with the opinions expressed by the commentators?

Each critical incident and its commentaries forms an independent unit that is intended to be read, pondered, and discussed. The reader should feel free to read the incidents in any order he or she sees fit. However, for convenience, the incidents are grouped into four sections. The section entitled "The Physician in Training" includes incidents that deal with subjects relating to the training of family physicians. The section entitled "The Professionals" includes incidents bearing on the relationship between family physicians, the relationship between family physicians and their consultants, and the relationship between family physicians and nonphysician professionals. The section entitled "The Patient" deals with issues between the physician and the patient. It includes such areas as death and dying and the problem patient. The section entitled "The Practice" deals with broad issues relevant to the management of a practice, as well as ethical and legal issues.

The groupings of the incidents into sections was difficult and often somewhat arbitrary. One reason for this was the fact that many incidents related to several topics. For example, a given incident may have involved a resident physician dealing with a dying patient and a problem of confidentiality. In such a case, the incident was placed in the section that represented the primary issue that it raised. Due to the large number of incidents that encompass multiple issues, an index of the issues presented, which may be helpful if you are interested in a particular subject, can be found on page 267.

We hope that this book will be of considerable interest and value to you personally and professionally. The book can also serve as a discussion guide for medical seminars. This would be especially useful for physicians in training, to help them anticipate and plan management of future critical incidents, clarify their values relevant to the issues, and develop an emotional support system. In the seminars, the incidents and the commentaries can serve as stimulus for further analysis and discussion. Frequently, the discussion will include the group members' own associated critical incidents. Thus, group members can contribute, comment on, and discuss their management of situations that they classify as critical incidents.

Request for Additional Critical Incidents

As we explained in the Introduction, we are hoping to publish a second volume of *Critical Issues in Family Practice: Cases and Commentaries*. We invite you to submit reports of critical incidents based on your professional experience. Please note that we ensure confidentiality and that contributors will have the option of declining to appear in the list of contributors in any future publication.

We define a critical incident as an interpersonal situation that one encounters through one's professional roles or responsibilities as a physician, and which arouses either feelings of uncertainty about the proper course of action or feelings of discomfort, such as frustration or anxiety. If you would like to submit your own critical incident for possible future publication with commentary, please contact us at the address listed below and we will send you further information and guidelines.

Critical Incidents Project
Department of Family Medicine
Medical College of Ohio
C.S. #10008
Toledo, Ohio 43699

I / The Physician in Training

The many dimensions of family practice are currently being explored. The Virginia and other studies have investigated the practice content areas of the discipline. Various commentators and researchers are analyzing the process of family practice, exploring the entry into the health care system, the continuing relationship, the comprehensive approach, and the focus upon the family unit. While many observers have examined the role of the physician and the reactions of physicians to stress, a self and peer exploration has not been previously recorded.

Critical Issues in Family Practice is an exploration of the personal experiences of family practice residents and physicians to document their feelings and reactions to situations which are difficult to handle. The common themes for all physicians are highlighted by the selected critical incidents. Our commentaries utilize the collective wisdom of physicians and other professionals in considering the issues raised by the incidents. By sharing collective experience we are building a body of knowledge concerning situations which commonly affect physicians in training and in daily practice.

In a sense our book is a pioneer in the field of family practice. What Balint accomplished in England by working with a small group of general practitioners discussing together their reactions to their professional lives, we hope to achieve with you, the reader, as a member of our encounter group, using this

1

book as a national forum. The book provides group introspection, support, and critical commentary with an ultimate aim of better patient care and physician well-being.

The specialty of family practice is by its very nature complex. No other medical specialty combines such a broad knowledge base, a high degree of uncertainty, and a working relationship with so many other medical specialists. This complexity gives rise to common and unique stresses beginning in the residency training period and continuing throughout the career of the family practitioner. For this reason we were not surprised to discover that many of our incidents were submitted by family practice residents and by faculty members writing about residency training. In this section you will find 9 incidents and their commentaries that are representative of the important dilemmas commonly faced by resident physicians. Throughout the book there are other incidents involving residents' experiences, but it was our feeling that training was not the primary issue in those cases. Conversely, many of the topics occurring in this section could also have been encountered during the practice stage of professional life.

These incidents reflect the professional issues and personal concerns of residents in training. The family practice residency is complex, characterized by a unique, continuing experience in family practice and a rotational participation in hospital and outpatient training in other disciplines. These resultant identity, loyalty, logistical, and communication problems compound an inherently stressful period of professional life. These incidents are illustrative of the critical incidents in family practice training.

The Editors

1 / Mea Culpa
Patient Death, Physician Guilt

Background

I painfully remember the Christmas Eve of my internship year when I was on internal medicine rotation. The residents not on duty wanted to get away early for the celebration, leaving the hospital about 50 percent staffed. I was responsible for all medicine service admissions in addition to covering three medical wards and the ICU.

About 5:00 P.M., one of my colleagues wanted to leave and checked out his patients to me. He told me about a 19-year-old man in the ICU with purulent meningococcal meningitis, who had been in the hospital for five days on high-dose antibiotics. This morning's repeated spinal tap, done with much difficulty because of his great combativeness, again revealed gross pus. Since his fever curve seemed to be coming down, no changes were made in his therapy. I was told that he had begun to develop some fluid in his lungs but that no treatment was planned other than observation for the present. A chest x-ray had just been obtained and my colleague told me that it "looked okay with only a little fluid bilaterally in the parenchyma." I accepted the report without personally examining the x-ray. He was anxious to leave and reassured me that the patient would be no problem.

I grabbed some dinner, then made my usual checkup rounds on the wards. About 6:30 P.M. I wandered by the ICU to see what was happening. I had

3

been lucky so far; my beeper hadn't rung for an admission yet. I looked through the glass behind the nurses' station into the isolation room where Paul, the patient with meningitis, lay. He seemed quiet with his eyes closed but his hands and feet were in restraints. The nurses reported that he was pretty much the same and that he was stuporous and hadn't been combative since the morning. However, they were concerned because a recent bowel movement had been guaiac positive for blood. This concerned me since it was a new development. I wondered if he might be developing a stress ulcer and went in to examine him. His breathing sounded harsh, and he had some foamy saliva in his mouth which I suctioned out. I had never seen frank pulmonary edema before and I didn't think of this possibility. His vital signs were stable and he had no heart sounds indicating a gallop rhythm. Rather than focus on his moist breath sounds, which the nurses reported as a stable condition, I instead placed an NG tube, looking for an ulcer. I aspirated only clear fluid and injected an antacid bolus into his stomach before removing the tube. I ordered blood for typing and a CBC to see if there had been any significant bleeding. In the midst of thinking about him, my beeper went off. I left Paul to go to a phone and found that I had a new admission waiting for me on another ward. I jotted down the details and left without looking at the earlier chest x-ray myself, asking the nurses to call me when the blood count was done.

The Incident

In the middle of my new patient workup, I was paged and Paul's blood count was reported to me. There had been no significant change since his morning lab report. The nurse reported that his condition remained unchanged. Again I was lulled into a false sense of security. I finished my workup, then returned to the ICU because I wanted to read over Paul's chart to be prepared if any problems arose. I started to thumb through his chart, chatted with the technicians and nurses, and asked to see his chest x-ray. They directed me to a view-box and I flipped on the light. As I examined the film it became immediately obvious that his lungs were filled with fluffy infiltrates. Like a shock of panic, the harsh respirations, moist breath sounds, and frothy sputum clicked a signal of alarm in my brain. As I went to Paul, to check on him again, shouting to a nearby nurse for some Lasix, the nurse attending to him turned to me with a distraught face and exclaimed that his monitor was showing a bradycardia and his pulse was weak.

As if in slow motion, watching a catastrophe occur which I could not stop, I raced to his side. Paul had no heartbeat. I thumped his chest and saw pink, frothy sputum in his mouth. A cardiac arrest code was sounded. Then all hell broke loose as carts and people raced into the small, crowded room which was stuffed with monitors, limiting our space. I attempted intubation but his mouth was filled with pink froth which suctioning couldn't remove fast enough. An anesthesiologist arrived and successfully intubated him as we performed CPR. After a half-hour of futile, heroic attempts, Paul was pronounced dead.

In shock, the thought that I had killed him screamed in my brain. I forced myself to complete all the paperwork and death forms. Then I had the hardest task which I've ever had to face confront me. I had to tell the mother of this 19-year-old man who looked like a boy, so young and immortal, that he was dead. I was gentle and truly sorry, sharing her grief, but feeling the full weight of my guilt. I held her and felt her tears on my shoulder. As tears welled up in my own eyes, I cried with anguish inside. I walked with her to see the body, staying near her for support. Each shriek of her agony pierced my heart. If only I had . . . on and on, going over every detail in the chain of errors which led to the death of this young man. I was called away to other responsibilities and kept busy for the next few hours, functioning in a daze, yet supercautious, flagellating myself mentally for my ignorance.

In the lull of the early morning hours of Christmas, I finally sat down, numb and depressed. I wondered if I should quit medicine before another person would be hurt or killed by my errors and stupidity. I wondered if I would have that choice or whether I would be asked to leave my training program. I thought about Paul and his family . . . "Merry Christmas, ma'am, your son is dead." I grieved for her and thought of all the years of life he could have experienced. I cried, sobbing, with tears streaming down my face. I wallowed in my sorrow and self-pity. I tried out excuses without relief from my pain. I tried to focus the blame elsewhere or at least spread it around a little. Who had led me down the primrose path? Who kept reassuring me that his condition was unchanged? All this was for naught for I ached inside. All inside felt dark and gloomy. Talking with the internist on call and the other concerned physicians who had been helping with the case had been a mildly therapeutic punishment. There was nobody who could say anything to me that I hadn't already said to myself, and much worse at that. I couldn't accept the comfort offered by them. Questions kept recurring: "Why did this have to happen to me?"

Paul's autopsy showed "multisystem damage with destruction of capillary endothelium in the lungs, causing a massive leakage of fluid into his alveoli and parenchyma." The knowledge that diuretics and PEEP may not have helped and that his infection was so extensive that death was perhaps inevitable helped me a little.

I didn't quit medicine and I had no repercussions in my training. I received a lot of sympathy and support from the staff. My family gave me love and understanding. I studied hard, worked hard, and searched my soul. With time I forgave myself and grew to realize the very human nature of my chosen profession. I became more humble. I have tried to express my great love through my caring. Paul is dead. That is a fact of my life. I hope that I have learned, from this critical incident, lessons to guide me in my future therapeutic relationships. I'm still going to make mistakes; it is inevitable since I'm human and not perfect. All I can do is try my very best to be as knowledgeable, competent, and as caring as I am able. I must be flexible and continue to learn, and be gentle and forgiving of myself and others. Medicine is a hard road to travel.

Discussion

What do you do when you screw up? How do you live with the plain and simple fact that you aren't perfect and that you make mistakes? When you are a physician, the errors in judgment can be tragic. Sometimes the stakes are very high and if you misjudge, miscalculate, or miss the whole ballgame through sloth or ignorance, people can become injured and even die. Of course it doesn't take a big life-or-death struggle to underline your inadequacies. Your errors may be those of commission or omission. Each and every time that you become aware of your own shortcomings, it costs plenty in pain and suffering—the patient's and your own.

Commentary

How do physicians handle their mistakes? How does a doctor evaluate the severity of an error? Is death the only parameter? Are recognized mistakes the only ones for which a physician should be liable? Who is responsible for the mistakes of a resident?

Without excessive rumination on all of these legal and moral questions which can only be answered in the minds of each individual, the author of this critical incident has related several facts and feelings about the episode that make it so patently relevant to all physicians:

1. The intern was basically unsupervised by a senior resident or private physician at the time of the incident.
2. Although inexperienced in the diagnosis of pulmonary edema, the trainee was aware of the condition, could diagnose it by chest x-ray, and thought of it when presented with x-ray evidence after becoming aware of other physical signs and symptoms.
3. The intern, a caring person who not only felt saddened at the death of the patient but felt empathy enough to hold the mother, could cry and admit it, although it was done privately.
4. The physician sought professional and personal solace concerning the

grief and pain. While looking for others to blame, the feelings engendered were never addressed toward the other intern, be it anger, pity, fear, or all of these.

5. The intern learned the personal frailties of a physician and has learned to forgive him- or herself.

Medical student and internship experiences are not often complementary in attempting to offer well-rounded, complete experiences to physicians. The medical educational system cannot keep one from graduating because the student has not diagnosed and treated a case of pulmonary edema. No curriculum committee could ever finish a list of those things which they feel each student or resident ought to accomplish. Perhaps a few vital topics could be identified, but many unusual conditions would also be necessary, so where to stop is a problem. Physician training should be aimed at basic knowledge which can be applied. However, this thinking process of diagnosis and treatment is not stressed as much as algorithms, lab tests, and crisis medicine. Teaching by example and critiquing a learner through an experience will hopefully imbue some of these thoughts and processes in the learner.

Physicians are human and have a right and an ability to feel sad or happy. This can and should be expressed outwardly in a manner which is appropriate for each individual for a particular situation. Touching, holding, crying, and laughing may not be things each physician does by him- or herself. But for those who do, it should be a natural phenomenon. Avoidance of these actions may in fact be viewed by people as an absence of feeling.

A physician needs support systems not relegated only to him- or herself, family, or even other professionals. Yet some physicians are not even aware of how to utilize any or all of these. Being a human with normal feelings does not make one less of a physician. A physician needs not only to be aware of his or her family's presence but also that the family can be a source of solace. So can teachers, peers, and others with whom one is professionally involved.

Physicians occasionally are quick to blame others for problems or to conversely protect peers from their frailties and mistakes. A physician should be willing to receive some input from a peer and also should be willing to offer the same to others. However, just as self-blame has to be dealt with, so too the castigating of others must clearly be removed from the teaching process. Blaming others is not a learner need, but the ability to deal with another physician's mistakes is.

To forgive may be available only to the divine, but the ability to learn from one's experiences and to work through the guilt and fear and anger in view of the practical realities of a situation is a reflection of one's own maturity. A physician's progress through educational experiences in life is measured in the ability to deal with these experiences appropriately. A good physician is a mature person, and a mature person is one who is always able to learn, adapt, and act responsibly.

The author appears to have been a mature person or matured since the incident to a great degree. This is not for others to judge now, however. This incident is exactly one of those situations feared by medical students. It is part of the responsibility with which physicians who are involved directly with patient care must deal. For family physicians as well as others it may not only come in the hospital in crisis or acute situations. The death of an unborn child, the progressing cancer in an aging grandparent, or the deterioration of a chronic alcoholic can have similar, yet different, meaning. For in those instances it is not the mistakes but often the inability to do more for the patient which bothers the physician. For the family physician it happens to patients who have been known over a period of time. Then the need by the family for a personal, caring human as a physician is even greater.

Ross R. Black II, M.D.
Associate Director
Family Practice Center
Akron City Hospital
Akron, Ohio

Commentary

This case is particularly poignant because the first patient death for which the physician has sole responsibility is, in many respects, the ultimate growth experience for the medical doctor. It highlights the emotional aspects of the basic human issues of competence and death, which, while not unique to medicine, do have a special relationship in the area of medical care. The introspective recollections of that long internship night keenly describe the enduring conflicts of dealing with a patient's death, as well as the medical system's abilities and inabilities to support its practitioners.

The primary portrait that emerges from this incident is the collection of the feelings of anger, self-accusation, loss, and remorse as responses to losing a patient. It is important to realize that the process described in this incident is a normal one. The self-questioning and grief processes, although painful and unpleasant, are inescapable if the physician is to achieve a healthy and mature medical perspective. The denial of this process is apt to signify or lead to a physician who, in some manner, is personally or professionally impaired.

The perspective gained by the individual reporting this incident appears rational, integrated, and adaptive. Acceptance of imperfection (or humanness) by a physician is not always easily gained. This particular lesson was learned under difficult circumstances, in an Intensive Care Unit—medicine's ultimate shrine to prolonging life where, even if apathy and insensitivity have not already developed, death is still an anathema. Yet, philosophically, an adaptive understanding was achieved; an understanding that balances acceptance of death with interventive zeal while recognizing the delicacy of that balance.

The critical incident description also highlights several correlated issues which influence the physician's response to loss of a patient and the resolution of consequent feelings.

First, there is the question of adequate coverage and support by the hospital staff. One might seriously question the ability of any physician to adequately cover "all medicine service admissions, three medical wards, and the ICU," let alone a first-year intern. Despite repeated studies indicating decrements in performance when physicians or residents are overextended, inordinate demands on residents continue. Such untenable conditions suggest that part of the burden of medical miscalculations might be directed to the health care service and training system, although such incidents are usually seen as a personal defeat complete with all its crushing implications. Certainly, a total projection of responsibility to the "system" is neither healthy nor realistic, but contemporary conditions generally mean a system which refuses to accept any responsibility. Unfortunately, one major effect of having survived this training is an insensitivity in the graduate physician, which allows the system to be self-perpetuating.

As a second correlative question, one might also wonder whether the resident should not have made a point of viewing the x-ray himself and, more importantly, of consulting the attending physician or upper level resident. The issue raised here is the ability to trust the accuracy of the report of one's colleague. While this must certainly be judged on an individual basis, the prevalence of contemporary concerns about "dumping" or "turfing" patients suggests a less than optimum level of trust.

Flowing from this is the larger concern of comfort in approaching colleagues in insecure situations. While not clearly revealed in the incident account, it has been my experience that physicians often have great difficulty in approaching other physicians and other medical personnel for fear of appearing inadequate or incompetent. This behavior is apparently a residual from the medical education process and the "*New England Journal* Citation" syndrome of one-upmanship. Competition is certainly healthy and productive, but it must be asked whether in medical training and patient care it has become so brutally refined as to destroy the human fabric of its practitioners.

Another issue raised by the incident concerns informing the family about a relative's death. Next to losing a patient, this is the most difficult and unpleasant task for the physician. This may be perceived by the physician as a process of not only being defeated, but also of having to confess defeat. It is, therefore, not surprising, though inexcusable, that physicians will at times attempt to avoid this situation by delegating responsibility to the resident on call.

It appears from the description of the incident that this is such a case where the notification of death came not from the attending personal physician (where there was presumably rapport and relationship), but from a relative stranger to the patient and family. To be informed of a son's death by an unknown physician, who may have few details or answers to many questions, violates every premise of the doctor–patient relationship. Fortunately for the family, this incident describes a sensitive intern who, at his own emotional expense, was able to stay with the family to provide as much support as possible. It always is my recommendation to residents that, whenever possible, they insist that the primary attending physician inform the family of a death to minimize stress for both family and resident.

In conclusion, there are several central themes in this incident. The case is a description of the most difficult but potentially maturing process of the physician. This specific case comes from an introspective and sensitive physician who, after experiencing normal emotional turmoil, was able to reach a rational philosophical balance with regard to responsibility for patient care and death. The incident also suggests characteristics of the medical system and training which may exacerbate rather than mollify this difficult time in a physician's career. These include the ability or inability to trust fellow physicians, excessive demands for competition and competence, and unfair duty delegation.

It must also be realized that medicine is, fortunately, regaining its concern for the humanness of both practitioners and patients, a trend which has been led in great measure by the emergence of Family Medicine as a specialty. The use of group discussion and group processes, based on Balint's model, is gaining acceptance at all levels of medical training to clarify such important philosophical, ethical, and emotional issues for physicians. It is a sad statement that residents today are still regarded as only "bodies" or more grist for the medical mill of established physicians. To the extent that medicine can adopt the model of other professions, where young graduates are accepted as junior colleagues and accorded respect, concern, and compassion on both a personal and a professional level, new physicians will be able to live with their human limitations and to realize that death is a part of medicine. To that extent they will be able to give support to patient and family and, as important, give and seek support among themselves.

Michael J. Asken, Ph.D.
Director, Behavioral Science & Medical Psychology
Department of Family Medicine
Polyclinic Medical Center
Harrisburg, Pennsylvania

2 / Second-Class Citizen
Resident Status on Other Services

Background
As a first-year family practice resident about to begin my first clinical rotation in obstetrics, I was enthusiastic and eager to work and learn, in anticipation of doing a large amount of obstetrics in my future practice. However, it is interesting that in medicine, as in everything else, conflicts of interest exist. I had no idea at the time that such a conflict existed between the OB/GYN staff and the family practitioners regarding obstetrics and gynecology. As far as I was concerned, I was a first-year resident and wanted to do the best possible work. Having recently moved to the area from another city where the medical college did not have a department of family medicine, I was unfamiliar with the residents, the hospital, and the staff where I was about to rotate. I recalled that before the rotation I went to bed early with butterflies in my stomach in anticipation of a month of night call, endless deliveries, and hard work. All the residents on the service met with the chief resident at 7:00 A.M. the first morning in the OB conference room to get their schedules and their responsibilities.

The Incident
I showed up bright and early that morning but was not the first person in the conference room. I introduced myself to the other family practice resident who would be rotating with me. Soon thereafter three OB/GYN residents

introduced themselves, and finally the chief OB resident and the senior family practice resident on the service appeared. Also present was the head of the OB/GYN nursing staff and the chief of the department of obstetrics and gynecology. When the chief resident of obstetrics and gynecology passed out the schedules, I noted that my schedule was a different color from the schedule that he had passed out to the OB/GYN residents. I soon discovered that there were two schedules. The chief resident of OB/GYN explained that "because there just aren't enough deliveries here," and "because we have our own new, eager residents" the family practice residents would be limited to their own family practice clinic patients and the family practice attending deliveries. There would be an OB/GYN resident on service concomitantly with the family practice resident and he would be responsible for all patients of the OB/GYN attendings, the OB/GYN clinic patients, and all OB/GYN consultations to the emergency room and to the floor. The family practice residents, however, would be required to do GYN workups on private attendings' patients admitted for elective surgery. They would not be expected to scrub for surgery but the option was available if it did not conflict with one of the routine OB clinics. It was then that I realized that the obstretrics rotation that I had embarked upon would not fulfill my educational goals, as I had anticipated. The hospital in question had sufficient numbers of deliveries but the obstetricians had arbitrarily partitioned patients, overwhelmingly favoring their own residents' education and ignoring the needs of the family practice residents.

Discussion

What ethical obligations do the obstetricians and gynecologists have to the public in the teaching of family practice residents, who they probably perceive as patient care competitors, even though obstetrical privileges may be sharply defined and limited? Should we as family practitioners not do OB? Will our patients receive suboptimal OB care due to a lack of adequate training?

Commentary

This incident reflects inadequate planning and arrangements for an appropriate educational experience in obstetrics-gynecology for family practice residents. It appears that the "double system" of obstetric care and training described here will minimize interactions between the house staff and attending physicians in obstetrics-gynecology and family practice which will inevitably compromise teaching and learning for the house staff in both disciplines.

Not only have the family practice residents been excluded from a sufficient number of obstetric patients and deliveries, they have also been scheduled for substantial service commitments for workups of private gynecology patients without concern for their educational needs.

The question of ethical responsibility for teaching on the part of obstetrician-gynecologists is clearly open to individual differences and potential conflicts of interest. While it is reasonable to expect the consultant to actively teach the primary care physician in the course of consultation for individual patients, it is quite another matter to expect, on an ethical basis alone, the consultant to commit personal and department time, energy, and resources on a long-term basis to sizable programmatic teaching commitments to a family practice residency, particularly under the circumstances where such a program might be perceived as competitive with or in addition to existing teaching commitments to residents and students in obstetrics-gynecology. Since good teaching cannot be mandated, the ethical question is somewhat moot. The involvement of obstetrician-gynecologists in the training of future family physicians must be based on genuine commitment, with recognition for the positive outcomes of this effort, such as enhancement of the quality of patient care through education and enjoyment of the teaching process itself. A good teaching program involving obstetrics-gynecology and family practice will necessarily require an atmosphere of mutual trust and respect, enthusiastic acceptance of shared goals, and open communication on an everyday basis between residents and faculty in each discipline. It is the responsibility of the program directors and faculty in both departments, not the residents, to plan, develop, and monitor such an interdisciplinary effort.

Many reasons can be advanced in support of obstetrics-gynecology training as a necessary and required part of the family practice resident's training in the United States (Geyman, 1974):

1. Pregnancy and childbirth, as normal and important events in the life cycle of most families, fall naturally into the purview of the family physician who cares for all members of the family regardless of age, sex, or presenting complaint.
2. The impact of pregnancy and delivery on the family as a unit can best be recognized and dealt with by a physician who cares for the entire family.
3. Care of the newborn infant, including complete examination immediately after delivery, is facilitated under the continuing management by the physician who provided obstetric care.
4. A substantial spectrum of obstetric knowledge and skills is within the competency of a family physician with appropriate obstetric training during a three-year family practice residency.

5. The increasing choice of group practice by family physicians will provide adequate coverage for the family physician's practice while the doctor is involved in obstetric care.
6. About one-third of obstetric deliveries in the United States are performed by general or family physicians; board-certified obstetricians cannot alone meet the demands for obstetric and gynecologic care, nor are they distributed according to areas of need.
7. Family practice, as the broadest and most flexible field in medicine, has already demonstrated its capacity to effectively address the problem of geographic maldistribution of physicians.

Although there are admittedly some regional differences in the practice patterns of family physicians in this country, with less involvement in obstetrics and surgery in the Northeast, fully two-thirds of residency-trained family physicians include obstetrics in their practices, according to a recent national study by the American Academy of Family Physicians of over 3,000 family practice residency graduates (Black, Schmittling, & Stern, 1980). Over one-third of these graduates hold some hospital privileges for complicated obstetric care, and less than 5 percent of the respondents indicated no obstetrical privileges due to lack of training, prohibitive liability costs, or denial of hospital privileges.

Some studies have already demonstrated comparable levels of quality of obstetric care provided by family physicians and obstetrician-gynecologists (Ely, Ueland, & Gordon, 1976; Phillips, Rice, & Layton, 1978). In addition, one study has shown that family practices which include obstetrics comprise more minor surgery, gynecology, pediatrics, family counseling, and family care than those excluding obstetrics (Mehl, Bruce, & Renner, 1976).

Suboptimal training in obstetrics-gynecology, as in any curricular area, cannot be accepted in any family practice residency. Considerable experience has been gained during the 1970s which can facilitate the development of excellent residency training in obstetrics-gynecology for family practice residents in any given program and institution. The recommended core curriculum jointly developed by the American Academy of Family Physicians and the American College of Obstetricians and Gynecologists provides helpful guidelines for curriculum development and the delineation of hospital privileges in this area (ACOG-AAFP, 1980). A model for longitudinal, family-centered obstetrical training has been described as a useful adjunct to traditional hospital-based teaching rotations in obstetrics-gynecology (Lynch, 1978). A comparative view of the content and approaches for training in this area is afforded by a national study of U.S. family practice residencies reported in 1977 (Harris & Scutchfield, 1977). An interesting variant of traditional teaching rotations was recently described in one family practice residency whereby obstetrical teaching is provided over the full three-year residency period on a nonrotational basis through the use of family practice faculty as primary teachers with attending obstetricians-gynecologists readily available as consultants (Crow, Rohrer, Carley, Radke, & Holden, 1980). Essential to the success of any teaching program in this important area, however, is the development and maintenance of a long-standing, cooperative, and collegial relationship between the participating obstetrician-gynecologists and family physicians based on mutual respect, shared goals, and complementary roles.

John P. Geyman, M.D.
Professor and Chairman
Department of Family Medicine, School of Medicine
University of Washington
Seattle, Washington

References

ACOG-AAFP recommended core curriculum and hospital practice privileges in obstetrics-gynecology for family physicians. *American Academy of Family Physicians Reporter,* 1980, 7(7).

Black, R. R., Schmittling, M. S., & Stern, T. L. Characteristics in medical education? Some approaches to problem areas. *Journal of Family Practice,* 1980, *11*(5), 767–778.

Crow, H. E., Rohrer, M. M., Carley, W. C., Radke, K. F., & Holden, D. M. Non-rotational teaching of obstetrics in a family practice residency. *Journal of Family Practice,* 1980, *10*(5), 831–834.

Ely, J. W., Ueland, K., & Gordon, M. J. An audit of obstetric care in a university family medicine department and an obstetrics-gynecology department. *Journal of Family Practice,* 1976, 3(4), 397–401.

Geyman, J. P. Obstetrics and family practice: Conflict in medical education? Some approaches to problem areas. *Journal of Reproductive Medicine,* 1974, *12*(2), 59–63.

Harris, B. A., & Scutchfield, F. D. Obstetrical and gynecological teaching in family practice residency programs. *Journal of Family Practice,* 1977, 4(4), 749–750.

Lynch, D. A. Obstetrics in family practice: A model for residency training. *Journal of Family Practice,* 1978, 7(4), 723–730.

Mehl, L. E., Bruce, C., & Renner, J. H. Importance of obstetrics in a comprehensive family practice. *Journal of Family Practice,* 1976, 3(4), 385–389.

Phillips, W. B., Rice G. A., & Layton, R. H. Audit of obstetrical care and outcome in family medicine, obstetrics, and general practice. *Journal of Family Practice,* 1978, 6(6), 1209–1216.

Commentary

The problems posed for this new resident are a cascade of all that is wrong with graduate medical education. Some would claim that the responsibility for careful investigation of the organization and quality of a particular residency program should lie with the applicant—a presumably knowledgeable and sophisticated graduating medical student mapping out a career. Most would believe that the existing accreditation mechanisms operating through the respective specialty residency review committees should act to assure minimum standards, that specialty organizations should set overall educational objectives and outlines for excellence, and that these, taken together, should provide a "warranty" to the new M.D., just as medical school accreditation by the Liaison Committee on Medical Education assures entering students that all U.S. medical schools are of good quality.

The difficulties encountered by this resident included a hospital with which he or she was not familiar, no advance information on responsibilities, a one-month clinical assignment, no written educational objectives, and purely local in-hospital division of patient care assignments. The involved resident, disappointed at the outset, took a first look and saw an ethical obligation for teaching being blocked by hospital staff obstetrician-gynecologists. The resident's "Discussion" saw his needs unmet, and a specific agent at fault, but he or she failed to look deeply enough.

The Residency Assistance Program (RAP) of the American Academy of Family Physicians provides program criteria (RAP, 1979). There is also an existing Core Curriculum for Family Practice Residents in Obstetrics-Gynecology (ACOG-AAFP, 1980) which spells out in detail both the cognitive knowledge and the skills which should be acquired in women's health care by family practice residents. The document describes three separate lengths of time associated with three levels of graduate medical education. Three months' education and experience with emphasis on office care is discussed for those family physicians not planning to make obstetrics a significant part of their practice. Six months on "a structured obstetric-gynecologic educational program with a sufficient volume of clinical material" is strongly recommended for those residents who do plan to include obstetrics and gynecology in their practice.

Additional experience, specially tailored to the needs of the individual resident, but usually within the bounds of the traditional three-year residency, is recommended "for those family practice residents who are planning to practice in communities without readily available specialist consultation and who need to provide a more complete level of obstetric-gynecologic services."

One key feature of this ACOG-AAFP Recommended Core Curriculum is the emphasis on a *joint training committee,* consisting of equal numbers of obstetrician-gynecologists and family physicians. The functions of this committee are clearly spelled out: develop objectives for the particular training program, monitor residents' experience, and evaluate the residents' attainment of these objectives. With the existence of such a joint training committee, incidents such as this resident describes should not occur. Next, the responsibility for proper orientation and for implementation of a quality family practice residency lies, as it does in any specialty, with the residency program director.

Finally, while the program director's responsibility is paramount, it is the resident trainee who is the advanced student. A residency training program should be selected by each physician to meet the career objectives of that resident with the same care that an undergraduate college or medical school is chosen. This selection should include a visit to the residency program site or sites and—very important—informal discussions with residents already in the program. Written residency objectives should be reviewed.

Implementation of a quality teaching experience within established guidelines by the residency program director, and a match between student objectives and the program, should assure good residencies—and soundly educated practicing family physicians.

Warren H. Pearse, M.D.
Executive Director
The American College of Obstetricians and Gynecologists
Chicago, Illinois

References

ACOG-AAFP recommended core curriculum and hospital practice privileges in obstetrics-gynecology for family physicians. *American Academy of Family Physicians Reporter*, 1980, 7(7).

Residency Assistance Program Project Board. *Residency Assistance Program: Family practice residency assistance program criteria*. Kansas City, Missouri: Author, 1979.

3 / Double Bind
Conflicting Office and Hospital Responsibilities

Background

By memo my residency director had communicated my family practice responsibilities to the chairman of the department of neurology stating that I would have three half-days of patient care at the Family Practice Center and two hours of educational seminars. The agreement reached with neurology, as with other departments, was that I would be released from my responsibilities on their service in order to attend to my responsibilities at the Family Practice Center. None of the other departments at our medical school have residents who have obligatory office hours and see regular private patients. This outpatient education, which seems unique to family practice, is the core of our education. We all anticipate that in private practice 90 percent of our time will be spent seeing patients in an outpatient setting.

On rounds during the first day of neurology I spoke to the attending about my family practice responsibilities. His answer was curt: "Of course I understand about your Family Practice Center hours." He further stated that "As long as you get adequate coverage for your patients here, I see no conflict of interest." In addition to inheriting three patients from the resident who had just left the service, I admitted two more. One patient was a very sick, 64-year-old man who had an evolving CVA and required neuro-intensive-care-unit support with a respirator. The next morning the patient was sick but stable. Since my family practice office hours were to begin at 9:30, I decided to get another of my fellow house officers involved on the case. Neurology attending rounds were usually conducted at 10:00 A.M., and although the physician was informed of the admission, the progress of the patient during the night, and that I would not be on rounds because of my family practice office hours, there was no effort to change the time of rounds or presentation of the patient.

The Incident

There were two other residents on the service, a neurology second-year resident and the neurology chief resident, each responsible for three to five patients. I contacted each of the flexible interns, who were not affiliated with any other department, in order to arrange coverage for my patient. The story was the same from both interns. They could not cover me because (1) they were too busy, and (2) since they had "no clinics of their own" I had no way of "paying them back" for their services. I took my case to the chief neurology resident. He stated that he knew the rules but that his concern was the patient's well-being. He implied that if I wanted to learn neurology I would have to be available "like anybody else." He said that when other residents from other departments "rotate on my service, they don't go running off to their clinics." He also stated that if I decided to leave my patient and go to my family practice office hours, then "maybe you shouldn't come back."

Discussion

As a family practice resident I have dual responsibilities. Most of these responsibilities are worked out before I get to the rotation. Unfortunately, many of the other department chairmen, residents, and staff do not understand the importance to family practice residents of having a good outpatient family practice experience. Therefore, these conflicts of interest develop mainly when we rotate on other services. Even though the flexible interns would not cover because there was no "payback," neurology should have been more understanding. The family practice staff and faculty expected me to be in the Family Practice Center to see my patients. The neurology staff expected me to stay in the hospital to care for my inpatients. Thus the conflict. It was not a simple matter to resolve. I called my residency director and he talked with the neurologist, who then allowed me to go to my family practice office with the chief neurology resident covering. However, I depend on my subspecialty education to come primarily from the neurologists and their residents with whom I work. Since I had "broken their rules," they were reluctant to spend reciprocal time teaching me.

Commentary

"In advocating any measure we must consider not only its justice but its practicability," said Theodore Roosevelt (Morris, 1979, p. 130).

The first two words in the background information are "By memo." These words may be significant since they may be giving us a hint that the relationship between the two directors is less than personal or at least that the agreement between family practice and neurology is not optimal. The family practice director "had communicated" the family practice responsibilities to the neurology director. Could it be that the family practice director is telling—not asking; demanding—not negotiating?

The background also states that none of the other departments have residents who have obligatory office hours. But do they not have outpatient clinics to attend?

Fortunately, the incident above is not an everyday occurrence, but it happens often enough over the country that it is important and basic to the structure of family practice programs. The broad question is: Just how far can one person (resident) be stretched and just how "schizoid" can a resident be and still survive the curriculum design? This brings up the question of whether there should be changes in the curriculum to prevent so much disruption. Fierce rigidity on either side seems inappropriate and probably will precipitate many more such incidents. Personalities of the participants color how each incident is handled, but the more personal contact the principals have the better the chances for avoiding misunderstandings.

Now, to get down to the analysis of this specific problem, one could take a strict approach—a bargain is a bargain—and argue that once made, the agreement must be adhered to under all conditions. This sort of rigidity you clearly reject, for it is incapable of taking extraordinary conditions into account. It requires us to behave in ordinary ways under conditions that are anything but ordinary. Indeed, in the case at hand it isn't really clear whether there is an agreement. For a genuine agreement to exist, it would seem essential that both sides have the same understanding of what's mutually required. If you are my physician and you think you have agreed to treat my asthma for the sum of ten dollars per visit and I think you have agreed to treat my asthma plus my sinus condition for seven dollars per visit, then we haven't really agreed at all. Each of us thinks we have as we shake hands and say goodbye, but in fact there aren't any shared terms and therefore no agreement. In the case at hand, the family practice department sees the arrangement this way: the resident will be excused from his neurology responsibilities for three half-days and two one-hour periods per week. The neurology people, in contrast, do not perceive the arrangement as a straight release from responsibilities for those periods. Rather, they seem to see it as a conditional release—the family practice resident is free to go IF he is not needed on the ward.

"As long as you get adequate coverage for your patients here I see no conflict of interest." Whenever the resident is not needed in both places at once, there is an agreement binding the two departments. When the resident is needed in both places, however, it would seem that there really isn't an agreement—each side thinks it has priority. With no concurrence of understanding at this point, there is no agreement to observe or to break. In sum, where there is an agreement, the absolute approach seems too rigid; where there isn't one, concerns about breaking an agreement seem to be irrelevant.

The alternative to absolutism is flexibility. There are lots of approaches under this category, because there are lots of degrees and ways in which to be flexible. First, let's take it as given that we're not talking about *complete* flexibility—wherein every situation would be handled on an *ad hoc* basis as though no agreement had ever been made. Rather, we're talking about those unusual cases in which we might have sufficient justification to break a promise, to override the duty that would normally bind our actions. What sort of justification might this be? Normally a duty which requires us to do one thing is overridden only by an even stronger conflicting duty which requires us to do something else. To analyze the case at hand, I'm inclined to look at the assorted obligations the family practice resident might have. By doing this, one might be able to figure out which, if any, are important enough to justify overriding an agreement which exists between the two departments. Off hand, these are some which come to mind (Morreim, 1980):

Obligations to his current patients. Already there's a quandary, for he has obligations, not only to his neurology patients, but to the family practice outpatients whom he has promised to see as well.

Obligations to future patients. He has entered into a family practice residency program in order to become qualified to deliver a certain sort of medical care. Those people who will be the patients of his future practice may rightly expect that he will be competent in his chosen field. This expectation places upon him the obligation to do whatever is necessary to achieve that competence. At this point the question becomes empirical as we inquire just what sort of action in the case at hand (and in similar situations) will best promote his learning.

Obligations to his fellow physicians. Again he's in a quandary, because he has conflicting obligations. Clearly he owes it to his fellows in family practice to carry his share of the work load, yet he has that same obligation with respect to his colleagues in neurology, who are no less busy. (It might be suggested that he doesn't owe the neurology physicians his time during those three half-days of his family practice outpatient clinic, since that was provided for in the original agreement. This line of reasoning won't work, however, since we have already seen that the content of the original agreement is not so clear as that.)

Obligations to the family practice program and its faculty. As an integral member of a program which is serving him as a physician by training him in his chosen field, it might be argued that he has at least some duties to contribute as well as he is able to the success of that program—which would include seeing the patients who rely on him. It might also be argued, on the other hand, that there are reciprocal obligations on the part of the program and its staff to help him out of problems such as this and perhaps to plan so that they either do not arise again in the future or are at least minimized so that he doesn't become too "stretched out."

Obligations to himself. He may have personal beliefs about what actions are morally best for him to take in this predicament. He and his values may be done a disservice if they are ignored as it is resolved. Another sort of obligation to oneself could be considered also. The "flexible interns" of the neurology service spoke of their own busy schedules as well as of the unlikelihood that they would be paid back for their extra efforts. Perhaps one might argue that one owes oneself a certain amount of leisure time; maybe time for one's family and friends would be included here as well. While this consideration is not directly at stake for the resident in the case at hand, it may figure into his obligations to his fellow physicians: insofar as they "cover" for him, they might be able to do so only at the expense of obligations which they have to themselves and to their families and friends.

To conclude, we see that there are clearly two sides to every question. We admit that the growth and development of the family practice program depends on how well the planners can include such times and incidents in their thoughts. The growth of the program depends on the depth of understanding the need for flexibility in curriculum design that is experienced by all concerned in such planning.

B. Lewis Barnett, Jr., M.D.
Professor and Chairman
Department of Family Practice
University of Virginia School of Medicine
Charlottesville, Virginia

References

Morreim, H. Personal communication, 1980.
Morris, E. *The rise of Theodore Roosevelt*. New York: Coward, McCann, and Geoghegan, 1979.

Commentary

This critical issue is one known to many programs. It has been a grave problem in some institutions. As family medicine is becoming better understood, problems in this area are fewer and more easily solved. This particular problem presents the opportunity to examine the administrative, educational, and ethical considerations pertaining to this issue.

Administration

For decades young doctors specializing in a given field have spent one or more months gaining information and developing certain skills on other services. In most if not all situations, the trainee had no continuing responsibilities in his own specialty. The practice of rotating on other services is universal. No specialty furnishes 100 percent of the teaching for its newest members.

Heretofore the centerpiece for each specialty has been its hospital service, the care it provides to hospitalized patients. Specialists' offices and clinics were conduits for getting patients into the hospital and checking on them after discharge. This system was responsible in great part for the ambulatory care deficit this country has experienced since the 1950s.

In designing a new specialty to meet the ambulatory primary care needs of our society, a *sine qua non* was that the effort be centered in an office or clinic. To become expert in primary ambulatory care, one must gain experience in health care delivery in this setting. At the same time a young doctor must learn more about diagnosis and management of diseases. This is usually and most conveniently taught as one cares for hospitalized patients.

Continuity of care is a *sine qua non* of family practice, just as ambulatory care is a cornerstone of family practice. From the beginning, it has been clear that these essential elements in family practice must be honored. Thus, the core of the training is located outside the hospital and consists of following the health affairs of all members of the family.

The problem emerges: how are deans and teachers in traditional specialties best persuaded to permit modifications and flexibility in their routines which are essential if the family medicine resident is to have a good educational experience?

Experienced educators were careful to communicate the above concept very clearly to their deans and to their colleagues who headed departments and hospital services. In many places, agreements and promises of cooperation were secured before application for a residency program was filed or at least before the program was initiated. Where the format for family practice education was not carefully explained to all and accepted by all, such problems as described here are commonplace.

Carefully explaining that continuity of care is as important in medical education as in health care convinces most colleagues of other specialties that some time each week must be reserved for family medicine. Demonstrating our own flexibility by negotiating which half-days are so spent and agreeing to leave noon conference attendance up to the choice of the resident can help win support. If a more direct approach is required in a university setting, then the faculty member can be reminded that he is paid to teach, that family medicine residents must be taught by him, and that he does not have the right to renege because the resident is not assigned to his service full-time. Hopefully, such confrontations will be rarely necessary.

In some universities agreements were reached with deans without concurrence of department chairmen. In those settings where family medicine was not given department status, family medicine was not represented at department chairmen's meetings and there was little or no opportunity to explain the necessity for family practice residents being in the hospital less than full-time. Fortunately the 85 full-fledged departments of family medicine now in our 130 American medical schools exceed 65 percent and continue to increase.

The critical incident described implies that the educational requirements for family practice training have been communicated and accepted by the chairman of the neurology department. Later, after a telephone call from the residency director, the chairman "allowed him to go to the family practice office with the chief neurology resident covering." The behavior of the neurology staff and the chief resident before the chairman interceded and activated a plan he had already approved suggests that the chairman did not communicate to his faculty and residents the working agreement with family medicine. This places the neurology faculty, staff, and residents in a potentially embarrassing situation: to have the chairman intercede, use his authority, void their statements, and reverse their actions. Here openness and good communication could have avoided a problem and preserved the professional dignity of everyone concerned.

The family medicine resident certainly walked into an unfriendly environment. One wonders whether the problem did not exist earlier and those involved did nothing to resolve it. For a new resident on a service to have the responsibility to arrange for coverage of his patient when away is unrealistic. In some places twinning solves this problem, that is, assigning two family medicine residents as a team, one covering the other when either has responsibilities elsewhere. In this instance, the chairman of neurology had agreed earlier to the educational format presented by the residency director.

The matters of changing the time for presentation of the patient and changing the time for neurology conferences are suggested. Again this problem of only one doctor knowing and managing a patient must be mentioned and condemned. To retard the investigation of the patient because the family medicine resident could not be present disserves the patient and puts a pressure, even guilt, on the resident. Neither should occur, neither must occur. To change a department's conference time to accommodate one resident would likely be counterproductive. Prior planning could have avoided this; for example, the family medicine resident's patients could have been scheduled or rescheduled to half-days best suited to the schedule of the department of neurology. Since any doctor can become ill or have a need to be elsewhere, good health care requires that more than one person be involved in hospital care and more than one doctor be able to address problems in the ambulatory setting.

The critical issue indicates that the neurology chief resident knew the rules "but." He apparently chose to ignore them and required the family practice resident to "be available like anyone else." Had he learned the "rules" from his chairman or elsewhere? If he had, then he was electing to disregard that which his chairman had approved. By misusing his authority he thereby created a problem and set himself up for a reprimand. If he had heard about the "rules" from another source, then his chairman fell down in his responsibility to communicate with the chief resident. For a chief resident to tell any intern or resident to do this or that or "maybe you shouldn't come back" is rude and crude. At the same time he put enormous pressure on the family medicine resident, he put himself at great risk for embarrassment when the chairman intervened. The sad sequela for this is the unfavorable environment for future learning which is created by such comments and pressure, all of which is avoidable by good communication and openness.

The phrase "broken the rules" deserves comments. Here the rules seem to be the traditions preferred by the faculty and chief resident. Certainly the rule agreed to by the family medicine residency director and chairman was to the contrary. When the chairman interceded, the chief resident followed the agreement. The family medicine resident may suffer a continuing penalty for having dared to challenge a tradition and embarrassed the staff and chief resident. One can hope young physicians who have teaching responsibility have sufficient insight to analyze such problems, work to improve relationships, and refrain from "getting even." Such behavior is beneath our professional dignity. One hopes too that family medicine residents have the strength, will, and resiliency to survive such ordeals, emerging stronger, more committed to family medicine, and wiser about the behavior of their professional colleagues.

Education
Residents in medicine and in surgery learn to respect the expertise and working style of each other while in training. The same learning should occur with family practice residents and residents of every specialty. This sets the stage for lifelong cooperation in practice. Training together, learning about each other as well as from each other, is essential if family physicians are to work harmoniously with other specialists in the future.

Family medicine residents have a responsibility to teach other residents the training requirements of their specialty. When two or more types of residents are working together, they usually cooperate, help each other, learn from and teach each other. When they do not, then it may be that their supervisors have infected them with their prejudices. The combination of reasoned responses by residents, faculty support to the residents, and faculty to faculty discussions usually solve the problem. When the *sine qua non* of family practice is challenged by another specialty's preferred teaching style, the former is likely to win.

In some situations, the director of a family medicine residency program may have negotiated agreements with a department chairman but a section chief in that department may not consider his actions bound to the agreement. At least as often when there is formal agreement but no acceptance, comments are made which make the situation of the family practice resident very uncomfortable. Here a double-barrel action is useful, that is, the resident insists on spending his assigned time in the family medicine center and his director supports his action fully while he discusses the issue with the resistant faculty member.

The ability to communicate clearly is a praiseworthy educational goal for most if not all family practice residency programs. The ability to describe accurately a situation and follow that by appropriate actions is standard operating procedure in the practice of medicine. Though the situation is somewhat different, the same learning opportunity exists in the problem case presented. The doctor who knuckles under because of pressure from patients will live to regret his action. After carefully examining his position, the resident had a clear responsibility to himself to tell the chief resident or the chief of the service that during certain hours he had compelling responsibilities elsewhere.

This type of situation is excellent for teaching another valuable lesson in medicine. It is very rare that the physical presence of a certain doctor is essential for the care of a certain patient. The day is past when much of the satisfaction in the practice of medicine was derived from a false sense of being indispensable. The advantages which group practice offers to patient and to doctor have dispelled this. Patient care including adequate coverage for every minute in the hospital is so uppermost in most doctors' thinking that it is difficult for many to accept that the greater good results from the young doctor attending to his education first in most instances.

Ethics

The ethical implications of the problem under discussion are important. In this situation, the rights of several persons deserve consideration as well as their responsibilities.

First are the rights of the patient who was admitted for care. This person is not aware that a new specialty is taking its place in the hospital, in health care education, and in the medical profession. This person deserves good care and to be cared for in an environment not confused by quarrels and turf battles. If this patient is critically ill, then constant M.D. supervision may be indicated. If this is not the case, then the patient should not be used as a tool to serve the prejudiced view of one side.

The rotating intern who declines to make a trade-off because he cannot foresee his needing a favor is extremely myopic. He may have other even more serious problems if he has adopted this value system at his age and in this profession. If he declined because he knew the chief of the service disliked having family medicine residents on the service or their being there less than full time, then he has the opportunity to learn the bad rewards which follow being used by others or which result from playing up to superiors by such actions. The service providing the learning opportunity has a responsibility to tell all its learners the rules and customs which govern the ward, thereby creating an environment which invites learning and cooperation.

The chief resident of the ward should feel a responsibility for the adequate coverage of all patients under his supervision. He also shares a responsibility that those working under his supervision have an optimal learning experience. If he communicates his disapproval for the family medicine resident discharging his other obligations elsewhere, his reasons require examination. If his chief has not communicated to him the agreements made for training in the ward, then an injustice has been done to the chief resident. If the chief of the service communicated disdain for family medicine residents or their training schedule and implied he would be pleased if resistance was offered, again the chief resident is placed in an unfair position. Such burdens are sure to prevent any chief resident from succeeding in having all patients receive good care, all house staff do their work properly, and all learn optimally. The chief resident in such a situation owes it to himself to put the conflicts on the table, clarify the issues, establish working rules, and get the business of patient care and education back on the track.

Summary

The problem discussed above is much less a problem now than in the early years of family practice residencies. All of us have learned the value and importance of clear communication and the proper use of authority. We have taught our colleagues about the concept of family medicine, working with them side by side. We have won their respect by adhering to our tenets, observing high standards of practice, and placing education high on our priority list. As we have made a place for the new specialty of family medicine at the university and in the community hospital, we have been alert to the

rights and responsibilities of others as well as ourselves. Much progress has
been made in our first dozen years.

Hiram Benjamin Curry, M.D.
Professor and Chairman
Department of Family Medicine
Professor of Neurology
Medical University of South Carolina
Charleston, South Carolina

4 / Sh!

Responsible Communication and Patient Care

Background

I was a first-year family practice resident on my emergency room rotation. It was usually a very busy service, oriented to a high volume of patients with the residents serving as the frontrunners of the care rendered. Very seldom was there a quiet shift, but when it occurred, it was usually from 2 to 6 A.M. This was not enough time for me to go to the sleeping quarters, but enough time for me to collect my thoughts and to interact more with fellow colleagues.

It was during one of those quiet periods that a 70-year-old patient who was spitting up blood was brought to the emergency room by her adult son. The patient had had a radical neck operation to treat a head and neck cancer a few years earlier. Recently, a recurrence of the tumor was noted on a follow-up exam. The patient, Mrs. E., was examined by the surgical intern. We usually took patients in order but he would usually shift the medical/pediatric problems to me and retain patients that had the earmark of a "surgical" problem.

As I watched the situation develop, Mrs. E. was shunted into the surgical exam room while her son, Mr. E., was left outside. He was a victim of polio early in his life, and he was leaning against the door with both crutches under his arms supporting his crippled legs. I felt the need to break the silence of this lonely-appearing situation.

I talked with Mr. E. for a while. He seemed to be a very kind and gentle person. He and his mother lived together in a farmhouse about 50 miles away from the city. Although their existence was very limited, he constantly took care of all her needs, even moving her around. He showed concern that this might be her terminal admission.

The Incident

While standing there talking with Mr. E., we both heard Dr. A.'s blunt conversation with the nurses and eventually with the ear-nose-throat staff about her dismal state. Never once was the son invited into the exam room or approached in conversation by Dr. A., but all the while Mr. E. could overhear the discussion.

The conversation consisted of remarks such as, "Well, she isn't going to make it anyway" and, "Not much that I would want to do for her." All the while, to my knowledge, the patient was alert and probably heard every word. I took Mr. E. aside and made him comfortable and at the same time wanted to be apologetic for the circumstances. I also felt frustrated at being caught in this situation. Most of all, I sensed the extreme loneliness of Mr. E.

Discussion

What should I have done at this point? Should I have told the surgical intern to please let the son in on the discussion and to modify the blunt, dismal discussion that was being carried out in front of the patient? This incident created a conflict in me in regard to professional ethics. This was his patient (family), not mine. Was it just that his style was different from mine? Did I have a right to question his method of interaction? We were only halfway through the two-month rotation in which we would be sharing shifts, and while I did not want to be in an adversary position, I still felt the need to help in some tactful way.

Another question that occurred to me was, how much had I missed in caring for patients during rushed situations? Had there been more Mrs. E.'s that I had never noticed before and only noticed now because time permitted?

Commentary

The family practice resident's description of the loneliness of Mr. E. was in reality a description of himself. His identifying with and empathy for Mr. E. are obvious, but the real issue was his sense of frustration in not knowing what to do and having to make a decision by himself—alone. His discontent and anger at the surgical intern only helped to magnify this sense of isolation and impotence at a time when action on his part would be a good defense against these feelings.

All of us are faced with situations which require us to act in a positive way even though our education and experience are totally lacking in the specific area. The family physician, in particular, is faced with many ethical problems which are relatively unique in the field of medicine. The ethical issues which are peculiar to the family physician are the product of the unique goal of family medicine—the goal of treating the whole family (Bibace, Comer, & Cotsonas, 1978). This is a worthwhile goal but gives rise to certain inevitable conflicts. The family practice resident's statement that "this was his patient (family), not mine" is typical of the long-standing misunderstanding between family physicians and other specialists. Michael Balint devotes an entire chapter to the relationship between family practitioners and other consultants (Balint, 1957). One of the main themes of the chapter deals with the ambivalent and not entirely genuine teacher–pupil relationship that exists between the family physician and the specialist. There certainly is considerable ambivalence evident in this incident, revealed by the reluctance of the family practice resident to decide whether he is a colleague or a teacher. This is referred to as a "collusion of anonymity." This collusion leads to a dissipation and confusion of responsibility when important and vital decisions need to be taken, as in this case.

The surgical resident's discussion of Mrs. E.'s dismal state is typical of the abstract and impersonal way in which physicians handle human tragedies. The dying patient is not seen as a person and is not communicated with as such. Mrs. E. is a symbol of what every human fears and what we know we someday must personally face (Aguilera & Messick, 1974). The fact that the surgical intern was tactless and allowed the patient and her son to hear his thoughts of despair is inexcusable and should be dealt with directly. The family practice resident may be in an awkward position, but to do nothing would be a disservice to the fellow resident. The Hippocratic Oath requires that we teach our fellow physicians and, in fact, that is where residents get most of their education—from their peers. His informing the surgical intern of his oversight must be done in private or else the family practice resident is simply discharging his aggression by humiliating his fellow resident. An open, honest explanation of his observation will teach both of them better patient care and a better understanding of the human condition.

The other main issue of the critical incident concerns a perceived territorial dispute. Although it is an emergency room situation, the turf is really shared by the family practice resident and the surgical resident. The reluctance of the family practice resident to step onto the surgical resident's turf is a misunderstanding on his part, because caring for patients should not involve arbitrarily established boundaries.

As for Mr. E., the resident should console him by explaining in more kindly terms the specific condition of his mother. An apology at this time would be meaningless and only help to make the physician feel better. Mr. E. should also be removed from the direct situation where he could overhear the medical conversation, but he should not be excluded from being close to his mother. Emergency room care first should address itself to the care of the sick and injured, but concern for loved ones and their well-being must be an essential part of total patient care (Warner, 1978).

James A. Ferrante, M.D.
Director, Family Practice Residency Program
St. Margaret Memorial Hospital
Pittsburgh, Pennsylvania

References

Aguilera, D., & Messick, J. *Crisis intervention: Theory and methodology* (2nd ed.). St. Louis: Mosby, 1974.

Balint, M. *The doctor, his patient and the illness*. New York: International Universities Press, 1957.

Bibace, R., Comer, R., & Cotsonas, C. E. Ethical and legal issues in family practice. *The Journal of Family Practice*, 1978, 7(5), 1029–1035.

Warner, C. B. *Emergency care* (2nd ed.). St Louis: Mosby, 1978.

Commentary

This particular case, or critical incident, has aroused much concern on the part of a first-year family practice resident while on an emergency room rotation. This uncertainty could revolve about the standards for the delivery of care, interpersonal relationships, and ethical concerns.

Some of the worries that the resident might have about the delivery of care to this patient include:

1. A rational, critically, and terminally ill person can hear and interpret what appear to be cruel, hopeless, and insensitive remarks, rendered by a professional who appears to be inconsiderate of her as a person.
2. Such remarks most likely would injure rather than help the patient and her son.
3. The surgical resident-colleague was willing to act before determining the patient's perceptions or wishes about her illness, particularly in view of the fact that this apparently was his first contact with her. In addition, there is no mention made of whether or not he contacted the patient's personal physician(s), who undoubtedly would know much more about her condition and her feelings about it.
4. An apparently brave, handicapped, sensitive, and responsible son, who cared for his mother and gained much from it, was not consulted and, like his mother, heard cruel, harsh, insensitive remarks.

5. Haste, such as is frequently the case in a busy emergency room but not so in this particular circumstance, can result in careless decisions and harmful remarks.
6. Innocent, tangential involvement with a patient's family can result in any professional's being indirectly responsible for the quality of care rendered.

The family practice resident's concerns about interpersonal relationships might include:

1. Guilt by association, for both he and his colleague are part of the same system, and he, too, may have been guilty of similar behavior, particularly when rushed.
2. Fear of conflict with his colleague, the surgical resident. Perhaps a large part of such a fear might stem from the resident's background and attitude about evaluation. All too frequently evaluation is considered an affront or punishment, rather than being constructive or helpful. On the other hand, many times fair evaluation can result in admiration and growth, rather than conflict. An adversary relationship does not have to exist. At this rather early stage in postgraduate education, being assertive, not aggressive, might prove difficult.
3. The family practice resident can identify with the surgical resident's behavior in a crisis situation, where he might have felt insecure about handling such a situation that included active bleeding and chronic disease in a patient apparently approaching a terminal state. Perhaps discussing this problem with the patient and family would have made both the surgical resident and the family practice resident more uncomfortable. Being detached and authoritarian-like is a frequently used defense mechanism in order to avoid personal involvement that might cause additional anxiety.

The family practice resident's ethical concerns might include:

1. A realization that the action taken had been harmful, particularly to a member of the family.
2. One has an obligation to "stand up" for good care and proper professional conduct that will be for the patient's welfare.
3. He has an obligation to share his observations with the surgical resident in a tactful, professional manner.

What should the family practice resident do at this point? It is obvious that his concerns in all three areas require that he do something, for his standards, empathy, and sensitivity would not allow him to walk away from the emergency room and go to bed. The option of denial or avoidance would probably not be acceptable to him.

It appears to the commentator that a "middle of the road," very honest, straightforward, nonapologetic approach should be followed. The commentator's approach would be to sit down with the surgical resident, after the patient's condition was stabilized, and tell him that, "it is not easy for me to do so, for I have fears that: (1) I might disturb our present and future personal and professional relationships and; (2) I might be violating some poorly understood or defined professional ethics by interfering with your responsibility for the patient." I would describe the situation to the surgical resident as accurately and unemotionally as possible, pointing out to him the fact that the son had overheard his conversation and had an adverse, upset reaction. Likewise, I would mention that haste, the emergency room setting, or the lack of previous personal contact, plus frustration and/or insecurity may have made anyone act similarly. I would not challenge his clinical conclusions, which I would assume were correct. I would point out to him, however, that he had eliminated a very important ingredient in patient care—hope.

For these reasons, I would suggest that I introduce the surgical resident to the son of the patient, and that he, with or without me, obtain more of a family and social history which would focus on the mother–son relationship, their perceptions of the illness, and whether or not both of them had openly discussed the situation in the past. Following this, I would attempt to enlarge upon my information by contacting other physicians previously involved in the case. Once all of this had been done, I would try to define who should be the one person responsible for the patient's care, and then with that person and any others involved, sit down with the patient and her son to develop contractually a care plan.

I would ask the surgical resident about his reaction to my being involved in "his case" and commenting on the care that he had rendered. I would also mention to him that I would hope that in the future he would be just as honest and frank with me.

I would also suggest that if the personal physician or surgical resident did not wish to exclusively care for the patient and all her problems, that I would be willing to assume this responsibility while she required hospitalization, and that I would be willing to work in close contact with the person(s) responsible for her care some 50 miles from the hospital.

Some of the issues raised by this particular case are concerned with doctor–patient and doctor–doctor relationships. Is a doctor a priest who dictates or mandates care and is inviolate or unapproachable? Is he an engineer who talks about all the possibilities extensively and frequently in terms not understood by the patient, after which he asks the patient and/or his family to make an immediate decision? Should the doctor deal contractually with the patient and his family in order to intelligently discuss the pros and cons of a particular situation? The commentator's own bias, as a family physician, is that the contractual approach is the best one.

Likewise, in our collegial relationships, criticism should be interpreted in a constructive manner. Not to point out deficiencies is unfair, for it allows them to be perpetuated and result in harm and failure to grow. To allow this to happen frequently requires attitudinal change.

Regardless of how desperate a situation might be, how harassed or insecure we as physicians might feel, the one important ingredient that should be in every prescription is some measure of hope, delivered in a real, honest, appropriate manner. Frequently, just a "sprinkle" of hope is all that is needed in order to enable the patient and family to carry on. Being brutally frank with a patient might alleviate our anxieties, protect us under the law, and prohibit our being personally involved with the patient in an exhaustive manner, but it really does not prove very helpful to the patient and his or her family. Maintaining hope, versus being insensitive and cruel, represents the difference between a professional who knows the art of medicine and a tradesman, who might be a superb technician, but does not conduct himself in a professional manner. For those insecure and inexperienced with taking care of the terminally ill, it may be best to delegate this responsibility to someone else who might handle it more satisfactorily. Such delegation need not be interpreted as a sign of defeat or insecurity.

Paul C. Brucker, B.S., M.D.
Professor and Chairman
Department of Family Medicine
Jefferson Medical College of Thomas Jefferson University
Philadelphia, Pennsylvania

5 / Secondary Gain
Disability Determination Dilemmas

Background

I am a family practice residency director. While covering for one of my residents, who was away on vacation, I encountered one of his patients, who caused me a problem of management.

A 19-year-old factory worker was referred by his employer for the treatment of back pain. The patient said he had been well until he developed backache during the course of his employment but not associated with any specific injury. He had worked for his present employer for six months and had been doing essentially the same kind of work he was doing on the day that the back pain started. He was examined by one of our residents two days after the discomfort started, was kept off work for about a week, and then went back to work without apparent difficulty.

The Incident

Six weeks later he returned and saw me, stating that he had been without pain at work for a few weeks after the previous visit but two weeks ago had a recurrence of the back pain. My questioning revealed that his symptoms were not associated with any specific slip or strain at work, nor had he any injury in the past two weeks. He was now having increasing difficulty with insomnia.

He reported that he did not have difficulty getting to sleep, but awakened frequently in the early hours of the morning.

My examination revealed a very tall, reasonably well-developed young man who appeared somewhat depressed and who moved with apparent difficulty. He seemed quite worried about himself. He dressed and undressed with some apparent difficulty, although he was able to stand on each foot in turn as he put on his trousers in the standing position. None of the usual sciatic nerve tests was abnormal. He was reluctant to bend forward, although his lumbar curve reversed normally as he attempted to touch the floor with his fingertips. He did not, however, bend enough to get his fingertips less than two feet from the floor.

Further questioning revealed that this young man had been "forced out of school" at age 16 because of dyslexia and poor school performance. Presently he lives with his girlfriend and their five-month-old baby in the girlfriend's parents' home. He stated that he plans to get married as soon as he has enough money. Back pain was a common finding in the family history with both of the patient's parents and the girlfriend's mother also experiencing chronic back problems. The father's disability was work-related.

My assessment was that this patient's backache was caused by a complex mixture of physical and phychological elements. I did not feel that he was lying or consciously exaggerating. My impression was that if the workmen's disability law were interpreted narrowly, this would not be considered a work-related problem since there was no specific injury reported by the patient. I felt that the patient was under great pressure regarding his present and forthcoming family obligations and that he was depressed. I thought it was interesting that three of the significant older adults in his life suffered chronic back problems and that he had been a "loser" since he left school at age 16. My assessment was that he probably had a mild muscular backache with associated anxiety and depression.

Discussion

The ethical problem arose as to whether this should or should not be considered a work-related problem. If I had followed state law strictly, it clearly was not. I felt, however, that he was no less a work-related problem than many other people presently getting compensation. We would probably lose him as a patient and lose the opportunity to help with this very difficult problem if we started charging him as a private patient. Therefore, with mixed feelings, I certified this a work-related problem and started a series of visits with management including large doses of salicylates, encouragement, tricyclic antidepressants, and hopefully in time some insight therapy.

Commentary

This case illustrates a number of important questions and issues that face the family physician. The first problem that one encounters is covering for another physician while he is on vacation. One is faced often with insufficient information to make the many decisions that are requested, in particular, in this case the diagnosis and acute treatment for an individual with back pain. This pain was sufficient to keep the individual out of work. There was also a question raised as to whether it was related to work injury or at least whether it was related to work stress. The issue of individuals requesting leaves of absence or sick leave because of pain is fairly common. Often the physician is faced with having to make decisions quickly that are personally unacceptable because of his own feelings about working versus not working. In addition, the issue of the physician's attitude toward compensation is clearly depicted.

The problem is further complicated because of the difficulty of making a primary diagnosis in many of these syndromes where pain persists but "no organic pathology" can be found. In this particular case, the presence of associated difficulty in sleeping with early morning awakening certainly raises the question of underlying depression. The conduct during the examination also seems to bear out this impression. However, there is not enough additional information in the history in terms of sleep disturbance, previous employment, previous history of depression, family history of emotional illness, appetite disturbances, physical complaints, and other information necessary to make the diagnosis of depression.

The information obtained concerning a family history of disability (both parents and mother-in-law) is certainly significant. However, by itself it certainly does not prove that the individual has the desire for disability and compensation. The past history of difficulty in school with dyslexia and poor school performance certainly goes along with underlying characterologic problems and difficulty in adjusting and coping, raising the question certainly of whether or not difficulty at work at the present time is really another episode in continuous adjustment and coping problems rather than a new "illness."

The physician entertained the question of whether or not this was a work-related problem and felt that he "might lose the patient" if he did not entertain such a conclusion. Certainly the judgment in this area is open to a lot of question, for the examiner felt that the problem was not strictly that of work-related pain. However, he minimized or tended to rationalize that type of conclusion by stating that other people receive compensation for similar types of problems; therefore, he justified placing this young man in a "work-related problem" status. It seems as if the physician "leaned over backwards" to find compensation for this individual in order not only to keep him as a patient but also to deny his own hostility toward the patient because of his attempts to get compensation as well as toward people receiving compensation in general. These kinds of problems certainly come up commonly and often one acts on an emotional basis rather than a logical, rational separation of one's own personal feelings about issues of compensation versus the merits of the individual case.

In addition to the issue of compensation and that of family background, a serious question was raised about the presence of underlying depression and instituting therapy. As mentioned before, this is possibly a proper interpretation from the data at hand, although one that is still premature. Other possibilities not really discussed besides muscle strain, depression, and "loser personality" include conversion pain and malingering. The decision to treat this young man with antidepressants, muscle relaxants, and psychotherapy seems to be overly detailed at this time. There are situations in which a therapeutic trial of antidepressants is indicated when one has strong belief that there is an underlying depression to a pain syndrome. Generally there is need for more data to confirm the presence of depression, as mentioned previously. In addition, the type of psychotherapy is certainly not clear because the history is rather incomplete. A trial of muscle relaxants might be indicated before any trial of antidepressants.

An additional problem presented in this kind of case is that of secondary gain. As mentioned, compensation is part of the secondary gain in which an individual receives some benefit for being ill. An additional problem is that the longer an individual stays in the "sick role" and on a disabled basis, the less likely one can return him to a functioning basis, and in many senses the patient presenting with the pain syndrome (particularly of a relatively acute nature) presents more of an emergency. When the acute symptoms become chronic, the likelihood of reversing and returning someone to work functioning diminishes greatly. The fact has been stated often that a six-month period of time for a workup and treatment is a critical length, for if the symptoms persist longer the individual will remain chronically disabled. From my experience, this has been borne out in attempting to work with individuals who have long-standing pain syndromes; even though treatment for the underlying depression and other problems may be properly instituted, the reversal of the secondary gain process is often not successful.

In reviewing the case, a number of issues have been briefly discussed. The issues of back pain, chronic pain syndromes, and differential diagnosis have been reviewed. Certainly, in addition to conversion phenomenon for which the history is incomplete, the question of malingering is raised in the problem and is often entertained. I would agree that the diagnosis of malingering is relatively rare, that conscious manipulation in order to obtain a pension is, fortunately, fairly uncommon. There certainly may be elements of more conscious distortion of pain and physical complaints in order to obtain attention and approval from the physician as well as to be out of a work situation that was unpleasant. In this respect, further history as to the nature of the work and how the person feels about it might be extremely helpful in generating some prognosis about return to employability. Second, this case illustrates a number of value judgments that are made about an individual in which the examiner or the treating physician not only responds in a personal and emotional way (which, of course, happens with all patients) but leans over backwards in trying to deal with his own anger. Comments such as "the individual has been a loser," "comes from a family background of chronic pain," "he has mild muscular backache," all imply hostility toward the individual. Such hostility often influences the decision that is made. In addition, the question of whether the problem is work-related or not is relevant, although such decisions are made by compensation boards in the long run. The treating physician makes a recommendation based on his examination but certainly does not have to make the final conclusion. Parenthetically, the development of pain in the job situation is possible without injury, and it certainly could be a part of a work-related syndrome. The presence of associated family history of back pain and the presence of many disabled individuals in the family setting would tend to increase the likelihood of this individual eventually being declared disabled on the basis of such history.

Another question that is not fully raised in this discussion was that of who was going to follow through with this patient—the resident or the attending physician? Certainly the development of a different form of therapy while covering for another physician is open to question in this case. It seems that the therapeutic plans as outlined in this case, however, are rather elaborate and certainly would be better done in conjunction with the treating physician as well as the staff physician. If there is availability of prompt psychiatric consultation, I certainly feel that in a case of this type, such consultation would be indicated before embarking on a diagnosis and therapy program.

The question of charging this patient as a private patient versus billing compensation was raised. It seems to me that the issue of charging here should be clearly the responsibility of the individual treated. The individual could later be reimbursed from compensation funds. Not only does this place the physician off the level of determining whether or not this is a compensation based "injury" but it also makes the relationship a professional one with payments made early.

In summary, this case illustrates a number of issues based on the physician practice, including the issue of one's feelings toward compensation, dealing with individuals that one has negative feelings about, covering for other physicians in their absence, making judgments as to the basis of compensation (whether it is indicated or not), the role of secondary gain, the question of making a differential diagnosis of pain including underlying depression, managing patients in a social, psychological and biological fashion, the question of paying medical costs which are involved, and finally the overall major issue of the best medical management of a patient presenting with pain syndromes so as to minimize eventual disability and decreased function and to maximize recovery and rehabilitation.

Marvin E. Gottlieb, M.D.
Associate Professor of Psychiatry
Medical College of Ohio at Toledo
Toledo, Ohio

Suggested Readings

Abram, H. S. *Basic psychiatry for the primary care physician*. New York: Brown Publishing Company, 1976.

Usden, G., & Lewis, J. M. *Psychiatry in general medical practice*. New York: McGraw-Hill, 1979.

Wittkower, E. D. & Warnes, H. *Psychosomatic medicine: Its clinical applications*. New York: Harper and Row, 1977.

Commentary

The obvious and most difficult question raised by the physician in the critical incident is whether or not this is a work-related problem. This, as in most Workers' Compensation cases, is vague with no obvious history of back injury. In addition, this patient has severe psychosocial problems which further complicate the situation.

The physician admits that if he would have strictly followed the state law, this clearly would not have been a work-related problem. However, if he considered it work-related, the patient would receive benefits from the Bureau of Workers' Compensation. The physician felt that not receiving such benefits would jeopardize further patient management and treatment with increased risk of losing him as a patient. As a physician practicing in Ohio, I would abide by the current Ohio Bureau rules, which state that

> the Bureau reimburses only those medical bills that pertain to recognized and allowed injuries and conditions . . . the Bureau insures only those injuries and conditions which occur in the course of and arise out of the disabled worker's employment . . . even then, the Bureau can reimburse only for those injuries and conditions that are defined on a claim application . . . the Bureau cannot reimburse for health care treatment of injuries and conditions that are not work-related nor can it reimburse for those that are work-related if they have not been defined on a claim application so that they can be recognized [*Ohio State Medical Journal*, 1979, p. 85].

The ethical issue raised is whether the physician can liberally interpret this law to state that his patient's signs and symptoms are the result of work. This places a tremendous burden on the physician and his conscience since the history was somewhat vague. No consideration is given that this may be partially work-related and partially secondary to other aggravating factors. To compound the issue further this is not his regular patient. It is unclear to me whether a decision had to have been made immediately or if it could have waited until the regular physician returned from vacation. As a residency director I would have chosen the latter alternative if that were feasible. In addition, it is not known what type of work the patient does, which would have obvious importance for the final decision.

The physician decided to certify this as a work-related problem for two reasons. First, he felt that this was no less a work-related problem than those of many other people presently receiving compensation. Second, he felt that he would lose this young man as a patient and lose the opportunity to help with his various problems. The residency director was faced with a "Catch 22" situation in that he must act in the best interest of his patient in giving him every benefit of the doubt while at the same time abiding by the specific guidelines outlined by the Bureau of Workers' Compensation.

I feel that the stated reasons are weak ones for certifying this as a work-related problem. From the evidence stated in the incident I feel that this is not a work-related problem. The history is extremely vague with no clear-cut documentation of injury at work, despite the patient doing the same type of work for six months. Since there is no mention of the type of work, it is difficult to comment on whether returning to work would aggravate this condition. As stated in the Workers' Compensation law, "all trauma and body members involved must be defined to the Bureau when diagnosed or discovered . . . even if involvement at the time seems to be of little or no significance . . . defining total involvement initially may insure patient's right to benefits if complications should arise at a later date" (*Ohio State Medical Journal*, 1979, p. 85). There is no mention of a claim application being filed during the initial visit.

There are obvious, severe, psychosocial problems in this young man's life. He presents with a long history of school and physical problems with the additional burden of financial, personal, and family problems and pressures. His forthcoming family obligations place a great deal of stress on a young man with low self-esteem. There are many secondary gains for such a person to be placed on compensation benefits. He has had firsthand experience in such matters with a positive family history of back problems, with his father apparently receiving compensation benefits.

We as physicians must be fair to our patients, to ourselves, and to society in such ambiguous circumstances and operate within specific guidelines as outlined by the law. I am sure the Bureau by no means wishes to be restrictive in allowance of work-related disability. However, if physicians recognize injuries and other trauma indiscriminately, the Bureau would tend to function as a general health care insurer (*Ohio State Medical Journal*, 1979). Even though the physician is often best qualified to recognize work-related disabilities, he also has the responsibility for recognizing those that clearly are not. Therefore, my assessment would be that this young man does have a mild, muscular backache with superimposed, severe, psychosocial problems and stresses, most likely accounting for most of the pain and thus not qualifying him for Workers' Compensation benefits.

Not granting these benefits to this patient could jeopardize the physician–patient relationship. This patient could interpret such actions to mean that his physician is an unempathetic, uncaring individual. To avoid such thinking, I would have been open and frank with this patient. I would have explained to him the Ohio Bureau of Workers' Compensation law to show him why he could not receive such benefits. I would, however, have made it clear to him that I was fully aware of and concerned about his problems, that his pain was not fabricated, and that I would do everything possible to help him deal with these matters. However, fully realizing the complexity and chronicity of the situation, I would be honest with him in offering no guarantees for an ultimate cure. A more realistic approach would be to help such a patient add quality to his life and have him deal with his own problems. This would be accomplished through regular office visits. If finances continued to be a concern, such office visits would be offered on a nominal fee.

Back injuries are a major problem in industry and a significant factor in missed working days. Unfortunately, most cases are in the gray zone with only a few cases involving clear-cut injuries with specific, objective signs. Many cases present with an unexpected onset of pain during normal, everyday tasks, as in this case. Some people believe that this may be secondary to local degenerative changes or conditioning from previous postural stresses which had increased the susceptibility to sudden onset of symptoms. This stresses the importance of a careful history since back injury may take place without a defined trauma. Many times pain may be delayed more than 24 hours after an apparent injury. The reason is that neither the facets of the apophyseal joints nor the discs directly receive nerve supply. Therefore, there are two major load-bearing tissues that may be injured without pain. With repeated injury these areas may undergo degenerative changes, and so what appears to be a nonaccident-related injury may be a culmination of a series of truly accidental, painless injuries that are all work-related. This is especially true in the unprepared, unskilled worker (Troup, 1979).

Falls, slipping, twisting, and being caught with unexpectedly heavy loads are frequent causes of back pain. Injuries are more common whenever the difference between physical demands at work and the measured isometric strength of the individual leave little or no reserve of strength. They also appear more frequently when the work load is significantly greater than the published tables of what is psychophysically acceptable in the population and the physically unfit (Troup, 1979). We, as family physicians, play a vital role in the prevention of back pain at work. Work should be and can be designed to be safe and to suit the population engaged for it. Many working conditions require unreasonable handling and postural stresses, which require a selection of the working population above the average tolerance to do such work. Therefore it is important for the family physician to be familiar with what the job requires.

The physician has a very important role in establishing the patient's rights to benefits in a Workers' Compensation claim. The Bureau of Workers' Compensation relies heavily on objective medical evidence to determine the patient's right to such benefits. The Bureau's policy of ascertaining a match between allowed injuries and treatment is observed rigidly. The medical care provider can be of great help to the patient not only in prescribing the medical care needed but also in assisting the patient in obtaining all the benefits to which he is entitled (*Ohio State Medical Journal*, 1979). This case is a classic illustration of the frequent ambiguity in Workers' Compensation cases. It also demonstrates the importance of careful physician documentation of injuries and conditions which occur in the course of and arise out of the disabled worker's employment.

George Darah, D.O.
Assistant Professor
Department of Family Practice
Medical College of Ohio at Toledo
Toledo, Ohio

References

Recognized allowable injuries under Worker's Compensation. *Ohio State Medical Journal*, February 1979, 75(2), 85.

Troup, J. D. Biomechanics of the vertebral column: Its application to prevention of back pain. *Physiotherapy*, August 1979, 65(8), 238–244.

6 / Triangulated

Patient Confidentiality and the Employer

Background

C. H. was a 21-year-old man who, in addition to working full-time at a local factory, was a part-time student. He had been a patient at our family practice center for several months for gastrointestinal complaints related to severe anxiety. When his previous physician left the residency, he was assigned to me for his medical care and to help manage his symptoms while he was receiving more intensive counseling for his emotional problems from our psychiatric social worker. I was amazed when I discovered that because of anxiety engendered by his heavy schedule and several stressful interpersonal relationships, he was taking both Valium and Librax simultaneously and additionally required several alcoholic drinks each night to help him get to sleep. He originally denied that his work was affected by the anxiety or the drugs, but it was difficult for me to imagine that these were not affecting his behavior. Later he mentioned some problems he was having with his superiors at work.

His past medical history indicated several "breakdowns" in which he broke furniture or struck out in other ways. In each instance he was brought by friends to a mental health facility. Fortunately, he had no history of violence directed toward himself or others.

The patient seemed to be very intelligent but had several paranoid features to his thought content. For example, he came to see us because he was afraid that his job and career would suffer if he were to see a psychiatrist and have that fact on his record. Family practice, however, was safe. Therefore, when he asked me to intercede for him if his superior at work questioned his frequent absenteeism for clinic visits, he specified that I was to restrict the information divulged to that necessary to establish that he had legitimate medical problems to explain the visits.

The Incident

While in the health center I was called to the phone to speak to the patient's supervisor. He confirmed my unspoken hunch by saying that C. H. was in trouble at work and was at risk of being dismissed if he took more time off for "health" reasons. I answered some general questions about the fact that he had medical problems and about the prognosis for their resolution. The next question was totally unexpected, "Doctor, do you feel that C. H. might be dangerous?"

I immediately felt pulled between giving an answer which I felt would be in violation of the agreement I had made with the patient about what I was free to discuss with the employer and refusing to answer. If I refused to answer the question, the supervisor would assume that my nonanswer was a tacit confirmation of his query. I felt sure that not to answer would have jeopardized C. H.'s job status even more. However, I felt that the letter of his permission precluded an answer to the question, while the spirit demanded that I answer it. Unable to think immediately of another alternative, I replied, "I have no evidence in his medical history of any violence directed at other persons." The supervisor then asked, "Do you think that anything we are doing at the factory is contributing to his problem?" In fact, the patient had described in detail a lot of his job dissatisfaction and how he felt that his true talents were not being utilized. However, by this time I had recovered my equilibrium and replied, "I would suggest that you take up that issue directly with C.H." The supervisor seemed relieved to hear that reply, said that he would do so, and hung up.

On his next visit several days later, I immediately brought up the phone conversation, told C. H. the answers that I had given, and expressed both my concern about having violated our agreement and my reasons for giving additional information. C. H. agreed that I had answered correctly and the matter was never again brought up between us.

Discussion

I saw this incident as a direct conflict between two duties that I felt I owed to the patient. On the one hand, my duty of confidentiality required that I honor strictly my agreement about what to divulge to the employer which did not include an answer to the question about dangerousness. On the other hand, I felt a duty to say nothing that would be directly detrimental to C. H.'s interests and, as he defined them, keeping the job definitely fell into that category of vital interests. My justification for my choice was that had C. H. anticipated that the supervisor would ask that question, he would not have hesitated to give me permission to answer as I did.

I also brought the matter up with my residency director and asked him how he would have handled the incident. He said he would have replied with, "Why would you ask a question like that?" This, he pointed out, would give me some useful information about how another observer viewed C. H.'s behavior at work and would also allow time to think of a more tactful answer while the supervisor was responding. Had I had it to do over again I would probably have used that reply instead of the one I thought of first.

At the time I did not think to question the content of the original permission which I obtained from C. H. Now, writing this, I realize that, should the situation arise in the future, I will probably be more insistent on getting the patient's consent to give more information when requested to do so.

Commentary

The principal issue raised in this incident is confidentiality in the doctor–patient relationship. As the contributor points out, the principle of confidentiality ordinarily precludes the physician from divulging information about a patient to outside parties, including employers, without specific prior authorization by the patient. This principle dates back at least to Hippocrates and most physicians view the protection of the patient's privacy as an important, almost sacred responsibility. In opposition to this principle, however, is the position that there are situations in which the rights of others or of society as a whole might supersede a particular patient's right to privacy. Examples include reporting requirements for contagious illnesses, gunshot wounds, and child abuse. Possibly relevant here is the California Supreme Court's recent discussion in the Tarasoff Case, which seems to place an affirmative obligation on the physician to warn the intended victim if a patient indicates that he plans to harm someone.

Another situation in which someone else has a right to accurate information about a patient's health status is raised in this case—the employer's need to determine whether his employee is legitimately absent from work due to illness or has just "gone fishin'." The physician in this vignette was given a release by the patient to discuss the illness with the employer, but the release was too restrictive. As indicated in the last sentence of the discussion, the physician now realizes that he or she fell into the trap of agreeing to tell the employer only what the patient wanted the employer to hear. "He specified that I was to restrict the information divulged to that necessary to establish that he had legitimate medical problems to explain the visits." Note that the wording is "establish *that* he had" . . . not "*whether* he had. . . ." As the physician states, the real solution to this dilemma would have been to insist that the patient's consent allow the physician to release the medical information necessary to answer the employer's legitimate concerns and questions.

Having accepted the excessively limited release, the physician was placed in a very difficult situation when faced with the employer's question as to whether the patient might be dangerous. He or she felt that there were then only two options: to answer the question directly, in apparent violation of the agreement with the patient; or to refuse to answer. The physician feared, quite realistically, that the latter action might jeopardize the patient's job status, as the employer was likely to interpret the refusal as confirmation of his concerns. Both of these options were unacceptable to the physician. Fortunately the resident found a way of replying to the question without directly answering it and yet satisfying the supervisor. This was certainly an appropriate and, in my view, an ethical action.

An alternative way of dealing with the question was suggested by the physician's residency director, who suggested asking, "Why would you ask a question like that?" In addition to buying the physician time to think of an answer to the question, this response has the merit of potentially providing the physician with useful information about the patient's actions in the work place and the supervisor's assessment of him as an employee. Another alternative, which would have enabled the physician to buy even more time, would have been to tell the employer that it is his or her policy not to discuss work absence certification verbally, but to respond to such questions only in writing and to request that the employer mail his questions to the physician. This would provide the physician ample opportunity to develop an appropriate response, enlisting the aid of the residency director or others, if necessary, and possibly discussing the response with the patient prior to sending it to the employer. The latter action might be especially appropriate in dealing with a patient such as this, as he is described as having "several paranoid features to his behavior." If the requirement of written, not verbal, questions were presented to the employer as the physician's standard policy in regard to questions concerning employee health, it should not raise the employer's suspicions about the patient.

The basic issue, however, centers upon the physician's responsibility to the patient in terms of maintenance of confidentiality versus the physician's right, sometimes overlooked by patients, not to be placed in a situation of having to lie to the employer. Had the physician insisted on a less restrictive release from the patient, a response to the question about the potential for dangerous behavior would have posed less difficulty. Of course, as the psychiatric literature makes abundantly clear, it is frequently not possible for the physician to predict whether a patient is likely to be dangerous. This difficulty is compounded in this case, as the physician had apparently seen the patient for only one visit and did not have enough information on which to base a valid response. According to the case description, the physician had only the patient's own story that the violent outbursts had always been directed at inanimate objects, rather than people. It may be that the employer was asking the question based on violent outbursts by the patient directed at individuals in the plant or other aggressive behavior. Thus, the residency director's suggested response to the question about dangerousness, "Why do you ask that?", might have provided vital information, both for answering the question and for use in the patient's ongoing treatment. Personally, I tend to be somewhat suspicious of this patient's veracity, as he displays many of the cardinal traits of the antisocial personality disorder, including work difficulty, irritable aggressive behavior, and failure to perform at one's level of ability. In particular, the patient's action in placing the physician in a most invidious position by requiring that the physician restrict the information divulged to that necessary to establish that he had legitimate medical problems is suspect. In essence, he required that the physician give only the answers he wanted given, no matter what answer the facts might dictate.

Regardless, the best way of preventing such problems is to examine critically any restrictions a patient places upon you when authorizing release of information, especially considering how they might limit you if the facts are not favorable to the patient's case, such as when the patient is medically ready to return to work, but doesn't agree with the decision or appointed time. This, combined with a policy of dealing with employers only in writing, should prevent problems such as that described here. The latter policy also provides the physician with documentation of what information he conveyed to the employer, both for the patient to see and for protection should legal problems arise in the employer–employee relationship.

Clinton H. Toewe, II, M.D.
Professor
Department of Family Medicine
Eastern Virginia Medical School
Norfolk, Virginia

Commentary

When the employer called the physician concerning the patient's medical problems, the employer asked two separate questions. The problem arises with the response to the first question. The latter question, concerning whether or not the problem was job-related, was answered by the resident quite properly and satisfactorily.

Without forethought, the question concerning the patient being dangerous would be difficult to respond to in a manner different from what was done by the physician. This, in fact, makes the physician liable and breaks the confidentiality of the physician–patient relationship. All states have laws concerning physician–patient confidentiality and the laws in most states are very specific on this point (Ohio Revised Code). The only situations that supersede the physician–patient relationship and confidentiality are those of child abuse, epilepsy in some states, reportable communicable diseases, and Workers' Compensation cases and cases when a person is in danger of receiving bodily harm (*Tarasoff* v. *Regents of the University of California*, 1976).

The response suggested by the program director is quite appropriate and does give the resident time to consider an answer, but he still has to make the final decision to break the confidentiality or not to give additional information. The patient has insisted upon this response concerning the content of the medical record. But the patient described in the protocol seems very unstable and could change his mind at any time. I am personally uncomfortable with a patient who sets limits as to the type of treatment that he will accept and makes the physician responsible for the outcome. I would have to establish more specific guidelines to work effectively with this patient. It is obvious that the patient has manipulated the previous physician into giving him drugs to treat problems that probably include alcoholism. The patient is requesting that the physician state that the problems are medical in nature despite the fact that the employer called concerning the safety of the patient and of employees around him.

There seemed to be a lack of communication between the employer and the employee. The employer obviously had more insight than the employee was aware of or had disclosed. It should be pointed out to the patient that his supervisor seemed to have a different perspective of his problem. I personally feel that if the patient was to see a psychiatrist, it would not cause a problem at work. In fact, it might improve the job status of the employee.

This patient has unilaterally established the guidelines for the physician–patient relationship and has manipulated the physician into being responsible for his work status. In addition, the physician is not permitted to use the honesty and flexibility that are necessary to establish proper medical care for this patient.

A physician must be able to identify the type of relationship that he has developed with his patient to be effective in the patient's care. Not to understand the dynamics of the manipulative patient will create in a physician a lot of anger and frustration which he cannot resolve. If a physician is to communicate with his patient, he must present himself as a person who also has feelings. In the incident under discussion, this lack of communication has contributed to the ill-defined physician–patient relationship. In summary, the physician must identify the dynamics of this relationship and openly discuss feelings, each person's responsibility, and the objectives to be achieved.

Frank F. Snyder, M.D.
Clinical Associate Professor
Department of Family Practice
Medical College of Ohio at Toledo
Director, Family Practice Residency
The Toledo Hospital
Toledo, Ohio

References
Ohio Revised Code 2317.02; 23.511.
Tarasoff v. *Regents of the University of California,* 17 Cal. 3b 425, 121 Cal Rptr 14, 551 P. 2b 334, 1976.

7 / Residents Are Human, Too
Challenges to the Traditional Residency Lifestyle

Background

I am a first-year family practice resident. One of the reasons I chose family practice as a career is that I have had a long-standing interest in the social and emotional forces in people's lives. Unfortunately, this has also caused major personal conflicts or "critical incidents" in my own life. I have also become interested in what makes "impaired physicians," observing the structure of medical education while being an active participant.

The Incident

A recent incident involved a fellow resident who had come to me after a behavioral science lecture on the predictable life crises of young adulthood. In this lecture, it was stressed that many young adults get caught up in career drives which cause them to neglect both their physical and mental health needs. We were urged to take a preventive approach by talking with our young adult patients about major life changes, work stresses, lack of proper nutrition, lack of adequate regular exercise, the lack of regular recreation and relaxation, and the importance of family and other relationships. This resident (as well as others in our program) agreed that we are totally hypocritical in extolling the virtues of preventive health care to our patients while they can observe us and easily discern that our bodies are (1) exhausted from a rugged call schedule that is a "traditional" rite of passage into the medical fraternity and (2) soft and flabby from lack of good physical exercise and improper eating habits.

Also, needless to say, the patients should be encouraged to treat their spouses and families in a more humane and caring way than we have the time or energy to do for our own. In discussing this, the other resident confided that he had become terribly depressed by all these resident stresses in the past few weeks. He was very depressed when no one else was around and had lost all desire for interactions with his family. He was upset for not being able to live up to the image of a perfect, inexhaustible, self-sacrificing physician. He had begun to question his choice of family practice, and he was not able to enjoy his own family and his work.

Recently he had asked for a "sick day" off from work because of a true, organic, medical problem and had been refused because there was no one to "take call" in his place. After he had confided in me, we talked for some time and offered to support each other, because I realized that many of the same things were happening in my life. Realizing that he needed help and some time for his own personal health care, I urged him to be honest and forthright with the directors of the residency program and tell them all that he had told me so that they could help him. He did just that and came back to me to report these results:

1. A sealed letter about his meeting with one of the directors was put into his personal evaluation file. He became very concerned, possibly rightly so, since he felt such personal information did not belong in an educational competence evaluation file.
2. The director with whom he had spoken first seemed to understand his problem, but then did not offer him any time off to get physical, mental, emotional, or marital help and recuperation. What the director did was to prescribe a subtherapeutic dose of a medication "to help you sleep." However, he told the resident never to take it on the nights he was on call because he should not be sleepy when he needed to do his work!
3. He lost some of his faith in me because I was the one who had encouraged the "heart-to-heart" talk with the directors.

My emotional response was (1) guilt for not trying to counsel him myself, (2) anger at the director for seeming so interested in getting the work done that he would sacrifice the resident's personal health, and (3) disillusionment in a system where family practice therapeutic principles were for others and not necessarily for residents and family physicians.

Discussion

Should I have tried to handle the problem alone, by giving time from a schedule which is already overloaded, thus taking time away from my patient load, time away from the already miniscule amount of time I have for educational study, or time away from my already-cheated family? Should I have discouraged him from speaking with the directors because there is an obvious conflict of interest, even though they are the people who should be able to develop a family practice residency where we care about medical personnel as well as about our "patients"? At the time he came to me, should I have considered him a "patient" as well as a friend? Isn't this conflicting relationship contraindicated? Also, isn't it easy to project that using such a drug prescription as a "cure-all" for his problem (instead of working to help relieve some of the life stresses) might encourage drug abuse and/or further physician impairment later? Why are we not allowed as residents to practice preventive medicine in our own lives and be role models for patients? Why are we expected to perform inexhaustibly and infallibly? (Possibly we could do either if we did not have to do the other at the same time). Why can't we see that the impaired physician starts in that direction early in medical school, in residency, when no one cares enough to let us admit we are human, or allows us to be humane to ourselves?

Commentary

The issues precipitating this incident are realistic to any residency program and should be addressed up front. An essential part of the behavioral science curricular structure should contain a visible and accessible support mechanism to handle or at least give a point of entry for help to assess and then solve such problems as presented in this scenario. My approach is a simplistic, practical one without a great deal of procedural rhetoric.

Several major questions are involved here. The first one is an obvious ethical dilemma of a co-resident attempting to assume the position of therapist with a doctor–patient relationship. Certainly this approach could be fraught with major difficulties, not the least of which might be the loss of real objectivity. Being in the thick of the forest, it may be difficult to view the individual trees with clarity. This loss of objectivity negates valid interaction. I would have preferred that this resident seek advice from an upper-level resident. With early-on "team" assignments in the residency, this can be built into the system. This arrangement allows almost daily interaction with senior residents who have been through the system. When such problems arise, they can reflect upon their own experience as it relates to the problem, offer advice, or suggest that appropriate further help be obtained if necessary.

As a second point, the frustrated resident, hoping to be helpful, did the right thing in this critical incident by referring the problem to the director. However, it would have been appropriate that a behavioral science faculty member be available at this point in the crisis. Given the route this resident proceeded on but not really knowing the director's rationale or personality, I feel the approach as described was inappropriate. Whether or not an entry was made in the resident's file is in itself not the important matter. I feel that such circumstances must be recorded somewhere. It is, however, how it was done that is a problem, since the scenario would lead one to believe that it was with a negative approach. The director's treatment approach at that point and subsequent remarks would lead me to believe that this individual was not a real family physician! The treatment prescribed and the directions which followed are in conflict with each other. If he felt medication was needed, certainly a support system was needed as well and should have been offered. It would have been better for the resident, director, and program to refer this resident to someone else and await an opinion before any decision was made regarding the use of medication, continued support sessions, and time off. I feel the resident should be treated by the faculty just as they train their residents to treat their patients. The co-family practice resident's feeling of "disillusionment" with the information given is legitimate.

The comments regarding personal "preventive medicine" and expectations in reference to "inexhaustibility and infallibility" are germain. We hear it all the time. Again, I say there must be a nonthreatening source of help available when such problems arise. Certainly, these problems tend to surface much more frequently among first-year residents than those in the upper level. I recommend that situations like this be settled outside the director's personal involvement, being informed only, and that the director become directly involved only if the other professionals feel it is necessary and important.

As regarding the resident's query about "beginning to be an impaired physician in medical school and during residency" and a "humanistic approach" to it, I feel that the problem in residency is much more solvable than in medical school. I personally do not have the expertise to speak about the medical school approach, although I think it deserves attention. Rather, I feel that it should be mandated that a family practice residency have a support system that shows residents from the beginning that, yes, we do care and, yes, we will help; that family physicians are humanistic and sympathetic, even in the process of training residents.

Donald E. DeWitt, M.D.
S.S.M. Regional Family Practice
Residency Program
St. Mary's Hospital
Kansas City, Missouri

Commentary

I don't believe that it is exaggerating to say that this vignette captures many of
the dilemmas and difficulties of medical training and practice. It raises concerns about such issues as the fact that medical trainees and practicing
physicians are often taught to give care to their patients, but deny this to
themselves and their loved ones. It asks questions about the meaning of work
and of responsibility and how medical trainees learn to define their answers
according to the role models who teach them.

The above issues are relevant throughout the medical specialties generally,
as well as in family practice more specifically. Furthermore, these problems
can be associated with life at large, medical training programs and centers as
well as interactions among individual practitioners in the community. The
problem of this writer becomes where to begin amidst such a large listing of
the interrelated factors.

Perhaps it is best to start with the first question raised by the resident. The
trainee, feeling guilty about the result of the suggestion, wonders about the
best way to have dealt with the other resident. Should he have tried to handle
the problem alone and not suggested talking with the program director?
Should he have dealt with the other resident as a "patient" as well as a friend?

My response to these questions is on several levels. First, I believe that the
first-year resident who wrote the vignette showed concern and compassion in
listening to and sharing himself with the other resident in distress. At the
same time an awareness of the importance of including more experienced
others was shown by his suggestion of talking with the residency director. It
would seem to me that this twofold response from the resident was
appropriate.

The director's response was to place a sealed letter in the second resident's
personal evaluation file, to prescribe a subtherapeutic dose of medication, and
to deny any offer of advice or counsel. This kind of reaction, especially when
coming from one's "boss" and a potentially powerful role model, would seem
to promote in a subordinate person strong feelings of his or her own lack of
judgment, competence, and personal strength. Certainly one would never
again risk revealing such feelings so as to avoid any repetition of this kind of
humiliation.

This type of encounter also would seem to promote a sense of isolation
among the members of a department or residency program. Each member of
this kind of group might spend his or her time and energy hiding needs and
feelings from others as well as denying them to him- or herself. Fear of making
a mistake rather than natural curiosity and caring becomes the motivating
force in this kind of system.

Now if we add to this mixture an additional ingredient such as the fact that
medical trainees and practicing physicians are often described as perfectionis-

tic, highly competitive, and achievement-oriented people who find it hard to set reasonable work limits for themselves (Lief, 1971; Rhoads, 1977; Taubman, 1974), then we can see how the resident who confided in his director might respond to the above-mentioned reaction of the "leader" by redoubling work efforts and ignoring personal and family needs.

As noted in the beginning description of this incident, young adults often get caught up in career drives which cause them to neglect their physical and mental health. If we can assume that the resident in distress is not atypical, then he, too, has been "caught up" in these drives. If anything, in order to be accepted in medical school he has had to exaggerate his career drives even beyond the usual push. The system has rewarded the efforts in this area by accepting him into medical training and residency, but has denied the expression of interest in his own health or that of his family by providing no time for this in a typically overloaded schedule.

The special pressures on the person who is a doctor, his or her developmental state, and the environment that reinforces career needs and denies personal feelings are powerful indeed. When one adds the life-and-death patient responsibilities that suddenly fall on the first-year resident, together with easy access to various drugs, one can begin to understand why physicians have higher incidences of drug abuse, marital difficulties, and suicide than other professionals (Coombs, 1971; Taubman, 1979; Vaillant, Sobowale, & McArthur, 1974).

Certainly the program director in this incident, who put a sealed comment in the resident's file and prescribed a subtherapeutic dose of medication for sleep without any continuing contact and counsel, might just as easily have thrown a match into a room full of explosives. As has been pointed out by others (Shangold, 1979), people in medicine such as the directors of programs are often guilty of telling their patients one thing while doing something else with themselves, their colleagues, and their families. Such negative role models keep alive the disparity between the patient, who is "allowed" to be subject to human frailties such as fatigue, neediness, and ignorance, and the inexhaustible, self-denying, infallible physician.

The portrait of the director in this critical incident is not an uncommon portrayal of directors in medicine (Shuval & Adler, 1980). While my own experience in family medicine departments is limited, perhaps having such a director in a family medicine program is doubly discouraging to a resident such as the one described in the incident. This resident chose a family medicine specialty program because he thought it was "different" from other areas of medicine, which are not as attuned to individual and family needs.

While it is easy, however, to point one's finger at the director in this incident, one also must be aware of the priorities in medical training centers and in our society generally.

For example, our society has made the physician a very special person. Society confirms a great deal of status and financial reward on doctors for the ever-increasing amounts of responsibility that also accompany this specialness. Because it has been difficult for physicians to limit the kind of special treatment they receive, they have now found themselves expected to produce miracles routinely. This kind of expectation is also the result of putting larger sums of money into buying and producing more and better technology as opposed to hiring more staff, residents, and teachers, so as to diminish the stress of heavy work loads. Thus, the director in this vignette is only one of many others who in part have been shaped by society's expectations, priorities, and technological advances, as well as by their own personal ambitions and the real and unavoidable life-and-death struggles of medicine.

An understanding of the above forces can help all of us, including the residents in this incident, be aware of those factors in ourselves and in society that make us susceptible to becoming like the director. Such an understanding can also teach us to accept responsibility and control for our own lives and to be aware of the price we pay when we give up our responsibility to others. That is, just as patients are now being encouraged to become more of an equal partner in their own treatment (Cousins, 1979), so trainees and practicing physicians can work together to take better care of themselves. The residents in this incident, for example, can decide to organize the other residents in their program for a personal support group. In addition, a meeting with the program director, seminars, programs on the impaired physician, and a changed on-call schedule may be established.

This incident raises many important and complicated questions related to medical training and practice. In considering these issues, medical trainees and practitioners are also forced to acknowledge their own needs and feelings as well as their responsibility for the care of their own lives and the lives of their families.

Lane A. Gerber, Ph.D.
Associate Professor of Psychology
Director of Graduate Training Program in Therapeutic Psychology
Seattle University
Clinical Associate Professor of Psychiatry and Behavioral Sciences
University of Washington School of Medicine
Seattle, Washington

References

Coombs, R. The medical marriage. In R. Coombs & C. Vincent (Eds.), *Psychosocial aspects of medical training*. Springfield, Ill.: Charles C. Thomas, 1971.

Cousins, N. *The anatomy of an illness*. New York: Norton and Co., 1979.

Leif, H. Personality characteristics of medical students. In R. Coombs & C. Vincent (Eds.), *Psychosocial aspects of medical training*. Springfield, Ill.: Charles C. Thomas, 1971.

Rhoads, J. Overwork. *Journal of the American Medical Association*, 1977, *237*, 2615–2618.

Shangold, M. The health care of physicians: Do as I say and not as I do. *Journal of Medical Education*, 1979, *54*, 668.

Shuval, J., & Adler, I. The role of models in professional socialization. *Social Science and Medicine*, January 1980, *14A*(1), 5–14.

Taubman, R. Medical marriages. In D. Abse, E. Nash, & L. Londen (Eds.), *Marital and sexual counseling in medical practice*. Hagerstown, Md.: Harper and Row, 1974.

Taubman, R. Being a doctor may be hazardous to your health. *Medical World News*, August 20, 1979, *20*(17), 68–78.

Vaillant, G., Sobowale, N., & McArthur, C. Some psychologic vulnerabilities of physicians. *New England Journal of Medicine*, 1974, *287*, 372–375.

8 / Scared or Impaired?
Dealing with the Disabled Resident

Background

As program director of a relatively large university-based family practice residency, I have encountered a broad spectrum of residents with a variety of problems. The current incident took place at the beginning of the third year of the resident's training.

R. S. was a very intelligent, well-read, family practice resident who received superior to outstanding evaluations during his many rotations outside the Family Practice Center. He could quote the medical journals with the best of tertiary care faculty. He had been married for four years and had one small child who was handicapped but receiving appropriate training.

The Incident

During the past several months, the resident spent an increasing amount of time in the Family Practice Center. The faculty had become concerned about his performance since he managed patients with chest pain over the telephone by asking them to count their pulse and had been verbally abusive to other patients, especially those who called for medical care during the evening or on weekends. During the day, there had been several instances when he had been unkind with patients in his approach to the physical exam and his doctor–patient interaction. For example, a 60-year-old woman came into the office with a complaint of painful legs and was afraid that she had a deep vein thrombophlebitis. The patient complained that the resident had absolutely no sensitivity to her problem. When she objected to the resident's approach, he withdrew, stating that she had the choice of submitting to his examination or going home. The patient's physical and emotional condition left her no choice, but she did say that had she felt better she would have left and never returned to the office. She felt that the physician was insecure, lacked insight, was unkind, and did not demonstrate appropriate physician bedside manner.

The resident had had several discussions with his faculty team leader concerning problems of intellectualization, authority, insecurity, and anger. These discussions and been most difficult and had generally resulted in no change in behavior and only further distance and independence within the program. After temporizing on the problem for more than six months, the Evaluation Committee finally agreed that this resident needed to enter psychotherapy.

Discussion

Management of an extremely bright but angry and insecure resident is difficult. Clearly, the faculty and the residency curriculum permitted this situation to exist far too long. There are very real concerns about his medical judgment when he enters practice. How do we manage a resident who is intellectually brighter than the faculty? How do we promote faculty contact when resident insecurity, anger, and sense of importance lead to independence? Can we require psychotherapy? If he does not resolve these issues with counseling, should he be permitted to graduate from the program and sit for the ABFP? Are the six months remaining sufficient time to resolve issues of this magnitude? How can we identify and manage similar future problems in a more timely fashion?

Commentary

In his discussion, the contributor has raised six specific questions:

1. **Q:** How do we manage a resident who is intellectually brighter than the faculty?

   A: His intelligence is irrelevant and not an issue. Residents should be expected to have a high level of intelligence. The issue concerning this resident is "What is the proper interaction with patients and faculty?" Before resolving this issue, the faculty must make some decisions about personal characteristics and performance standards for the residents in their program. The faculty then has the responsibility for supervising and guiding residents during their training with these standards as guidelines.

2. **Q:** How do we promote faculty contact when resident insecurity, anger, and sense of importance lead to independence? (Use of the word "independence" here is perhaps intended to indicate premature or excessive independence or isolation).

    A: My solution to this situation is to schedule the necessary faculty–resident contact and see that it is accomplished. Assign one faculty supervisor to the resident; schedule direct supervision of the resident for 50 percent of his time in the Family Practice Center; schedule the resident to observe experienced family practice faculty dealing with patients (modeling) for four to five hours each week; schedule videotaping of resident–patient interaction for review and processing; and schedule a weekly session for feedback and ongoing evaluation of progress the resident is making.

3. **Q:** Can we require psychotherapy?

    A: No, we cannot require psychotherapy because that is a private and personal decision. We can say, "Things are not going well for you, and if you think it will help, we can help you to arrange for some counseling or psychotherapy."

4. **Q:** If he does not resolve these issues with counseling, should he be permitted to graduate from the program and sit before the American Board of Family Practice?

    A: The resident should be suspended and told in clear language the specific behavior that is unacceptable as well as the minimal acceptable performance required to complete his residency and sit for his boards. It is then the resident's responsibility to show evidence that he understands that his performance and behavior have been unacceptable and that he is willing to seek and accept appropriate help to bring his performance to an acceptable level. At that point, his suspension should be lifted and he should reenter the program on a probationary status. When he has met the requirements of his training program, he should be graduated and qualified to sit for his boards. Should he fail to meet the stated minimal requirements, it is obvious that he should not graduate.

5. **Q:** Is the six months remaining sufficient time to resolve issues of this magnitude?

    A: An answer to this problem depends upon how one interprets "issues of this magnitude." What and where are the issues? Is this an issue of one resident, the faculty, or the overall program? The issue here is clearly a program issue; the resident is only a symptom of larger problems. This resident could probably be dealt with in six months. The larger programatic issues which have allowed and sustained this problem will take much longer to resolve.

6. Q: How can we identify and manage similar future problems in a more timely fashion?

A: As stated previously, the problem here is a programatic problem; the resident is only a symptom of bigger issues. Future problems can be prevented by:

   a. deciding what the faculty wants;

   b. setting up unit policies, procedures and standards for the selection and performance of both residents and faculty;

   c. scheduling direct observation and other evaluation of residents and faculty;

   d. setting up specific procedures for determining when minimal performance is not met;

   e. acting swiftly and with authority to intervene with corrective measures, suspension, or dismissal.

Handling of the Incident

Assuming that a decision to enter psychotherapy is a private and personal decision, it is inappropriate for a committee to require that a resident enter into psychotherapy. Temporizing on the problem for more than six months demonstrates a lack of responsibility on the part of the faculty to patients, to the resident, and to the training program. A major criticism of the handling of this incident is the failure to study and evaluate the faculty, the educational program, and the decision-making within the program, and instead focusing on the resident who is the noisy surfacing of the problems.

The Larger Issues

This incident raises a number of questions about the discipline of family practice and the training of family physicians. There is no clear consensus regarding the intellectual processes, personal characteristics, or specific behaviors required to be called a family physician. The definition of the family physician and family practice has been clearly stated. Minimal standards and criteria of observable behavior practiced by family physicians must also be clearly stated. The family physician should be a true generalist, an integrator, and synthesizer, able and willing to deal with problems at the feeling level concerning behavioral, family, and social problems. The list is much longer and these few are listed only as examples.

The next question then deals with program requirements and program attitudes. Are the above-mentioned behaviors considered in developing the criteria for selection of residents, and are those criteria used effectively in selection of residents in our programs? Would we exclude a bright, aggressive resident such as the one in this incident for admission to a family practice program if he lacked some of the characteristics mentioned above? Are those same characteristics translated into standards of performance and used in the ongoing evaluation of residents and in determining qualifications for sitting for the board?

Other areas for concern brought out by this incident include physician personality and the emotional life of physicians. There is abundant data documenting the personal problems of physicians and their families. The medical profession generally denies this "occupational hazard" of the practice of medicine. In a residency training program, this could be dealt with by establishment of a faculty–resident advisor system, by conducting Balint Conferences, by establishing a resident support group, or by requiring a "family study" of the resident's own family. It is well known that the faculty's attitude and observable behavior has a strong influence on residents. All faculty members should be involved in a family study of their own family, serve as advisor if selected, and participate openly in behavioral science conferences.

Henry C. Mullins, M. D.
Professor and Chairman
Department of Family Practice
University of South Alabama
Mobile, Alabama

Commentary

The troubling issue of the impaired physician or medical trainee is raised by this vignette. The residency program director is faced with deciding how best to help an impaired resident while continuing to maintain a commitment to providing the best available medical care to patients. In such a case, it can be very difficult to juggle conflicting demands and decide which course of action is likely to be most beneficial to all those involved.

Before addressing the specific questions raised by the author of this critical incident, I would like first to consider some important background information relevant to this problem. The 1973 AMA Council on Mental Health Report, entitled "The Sick Physician," defined impairment as "the inability of the physician to practice medicine with reasonable skill and safety to patients because of one or more enumerated (physical or mental) illnesses" (American Medical Association Council on Mental Health, 1973, p. 686). This report, based on a 1972 position paper of the AMA House of Delegates, publicly acknowledged medicine as a high-risk profession. Various studies have indicated that fully 10 to 15 percent of all physicians suffer from one or more of the following disturbances: alcohol abuse, narcotics addiction, and psychiatric disorder. It is also well known that physicians, when compared to the general population, are disproportionately vulnerable to both marital problems and suicidal tendencies (Derdeyn, 1978–1979; Herrington, 1979; Vaillant, Sobowale, & McArthur, 1972).

The position taken by the AMA in 1972 deviated sharply from the previous conspiracy of silence and punitive attitude regarding physician impairment. Until very recently, physicians strongly resisted recognizing the existence of such impairment in either themselves or their colleagues. Feelings of omnipotence and invulnerability, as well as the fear of the stigma associated with exposure, contributed strongly to this denial and to a reluctance to seek assistance. Although these counterproductive attitudes have by no means been obliterated, the profession is attempting increasingly to identify and provide early intervention to impaired members. The AMA Council on Mental Health Report (1973) stated that it was the responsibility of colleagues to assess the extent of a particular problem and to advise a course of action if the physician in question did not voluntarily seek professional help. This document suggested proceeding to the use of formalized mechanisms only if more informal discussion and counsel proved to be futile.

Currently, most state medical societies have guidelines for dealing with the impaired physician. Their functions vary from recognizing an existing problem and providing appropriate referral information to reporting violations in standards of medical practice to the state licensing board if treatment is not sought voluntarily. In general, however, most societies attempt to maintain confidentiality and to serve as enablers rather than punishers. They emphasize early intervention with the aim of keeping the impaired physician in active practice if at all possible or, if suspension is necessary, returning him or her to full professional functioning as soon as possible.

In the case presented, it is clear that the resident's hostility and insensitivity have interfered with both optimal learning and provision of medical care. However, the extent of impairment is unclear. State statutes cover only those cases where a physician's disorder leads to a specific violation of acceptable standards of medical practice. The situation is considerably murkier when the impairment consists of less severe psychological difficulties or when the physician possesses an abrasive personality style that is generally inimical to a good doctor–patient relationship.

A thorough assessment is necessary in order to determine both the severity of the resident's disturbance and the factors contributing to his current difficulties. How long has his behavior been noted? The author mentioned that the resident in question was extremely bright and performed satisfactorily on other rotations. Were interpersonal difficulties noted then as well? Perhaps the stress on the psychosocial aspects of medicine which is central to family practice does not mesh well with this particular resident's strengths and limitations. After careful consideration and discussion, it might be determined that he would perform more adequately and derive more gratification from another specialty. Are current stresses contributing to the trainee's difficulties? We know that he is married and has a handicapped child, but we do not know whether he is experiencing unusual conflict or problems in his family life.

Gathering the information necessary to conduct a thorough evaluation raises still other troubling questions regarding the limits of confidentiality. How can useful data from other sources best be obtained while still respecting the resident's desire for privacy insofar as is possible? Recommending that the resident enter psychotherapy presents another important dilemma. Can the residency program simultaneously protect the public and serve the needs of a troubled resident, or do these goals represent a case of irreconcilable conflict? It seems to me that these goals are certainly not in opposition if the resident agrees voluntarily to seek assistance and is motivated to resolve his problems. However, the author indicates that previous attempts to discuss the resident's problems directly were met with resistance and increased anger and withdrawal. I would wonder how these meetings were handled and whether they were experienced by the resident as threatening or punitive—consequently contributing to his defensiveness. Perhaps a useful approach would be to ask the resident how he would handle a similar case. In this way, his obvious cognitive strengths could be capitalized on in attempting a solution.

The author also asks whether psychotherapy can be logically required. In order to answer this question, I would want to know the guidelines of that particular state concerning physician impairment. Legal advice in this regard might prove helpful. There is some evidence that individuals can profit from psychotherapy even when treatment is entered involuntarily. However, it would be far preferable if resources outside the resident's own work setting were available to clearly separate treatment and evaluation.

In the discussion, the program director also ponders whether the resident should be permitted to graduate if these issues are not resolved. These are difficult questions indeed. In my opinion, successful completion of a family practice residency program definitely ought to entail demonstrated competence in the interpersonal aspects of medical care as well as technical skills and medical knowledge. However, I would want to know what criteria were presented to the residents at the onset of their training and whether they were explicitly informed that adequate psychological functioning and interpersonal skills would be required in order to graduate. Again, legal advice regarding acceptable criteria for evaluating noncognitive dimensions of functioning might be useful.

Finally, the author asks whether six months is a sufficient period of time to attack a problem of such magnitude. Although successful resolution is certainly possible within the remaining time, I would agree that earlier identification and interventions would be more likely to guarantee success. However, this goal is far from a reality in most programs and is an extremely difficult one to implement. The AAFP surveyed family practice training program directors regarding their perceptions of resident well-being, and more than 70 percent of the 233 programs that responded indicated having troubled residents (Coste, 1978). Few were able to report mechanisms for early intervention or, more importantly, prevention of impairment.

One approach advocated by the AAFP involved offering general support groups to residents and their spouses. Another group, the AMA Work Group on Resident Well-Being, is working to develop comprehensive model programs for providing support and assistance to help residents deal with the stresses of graduate medical education. This group has also made a general handbook available listing appropriate preventive and rehabilitative resources. Certain state medical associations have also taken the initiative in providing program directors with detailed information regarding programs and procedures, including a 24-hour hot line and interest-free loans for the individual requesting psychotherapy (Rosenberg, 1979). Part of the preventive efforts must also involve identifying those individuals who cope well with juggling personal and professional demands while maintaining a humane and compassionate approach to learning and patient care.

Ultimately, however, efforts at prevention of impairment should begin in medical school. A great deal has been written about the personality and socialization of the typical medical student (Cody, 1978; Funkenstein, 1968). Suffice it to say that medical students tend to be rather obsessive-compulsive in nature and to overvalue intellectual attributes at the expense of interpersonal and emotional strengths. In addition, the stresses of medical education, including the sheer enormity of material to be learned, the pressures to excel academically, the lack of personal freedom and time for family, friends, or leisure pursuits, and the prolonged dependency often lead to feelings of dehumanization, loss of self-esteem, and resentment. The inevitable discovery that the physician is not omnipotent is frequently accompanied by subtle pressure to believe otherwise. Faculty members often model denial of feelings and disdain for openly expressed vulnerability as a sign of personal weakness. One observer described this situation aptly when he wrote,

To a newcomer, one of the most striking features about medical education is the scant attention given to the basic psychosocial aspects of the socialization process, specifically the urgent anxieties that confront medical students. Scientific detachment and objective rationality reign supreme at the medical center, so that for the most part, recruits are left pretty much on their own to deal with their fears and inner conflicts. . . . Rarely can they talk openly about their feelings without risking being labeled weak or unsuccessful [Coombs, 1978, p. 134].

Many students, often finding their own training severely lacking in warmth and caring, later find it hard to give unstintingly to their patients. In addition, they may well be tempted to finally express, in a displaced fashion, the hostility developed during their long and arduous training when their low status prevented the direct expression of such feelings with impunity.

In summary, the seeds of this resident's problems were probably planted long before his third year of residency training. It is, in some ways, surprising that so few physicians actually develop emotional disturbances severe enough to interfere with optimal professional and/or personal functioning. Preventive efforts must be directed early in the process of medical education toward changing the attitude of omnipotence to an ability to know when help is needed. First, this involves an increasing acknowledgment of physicians' vulnerability to emotional disturbances both by members of the profession and by the public. Second, experiences must be provided that help students improve their skills for coping with stress. One useful approach has involved organizing support groups as part of the required first year curriculum. These were designed to help students adjust their expectations to the demands of the curriculum as well as to provide input that could be used in the process of curricular modification. The groups also served to sanction dealing with emotionally laden aspects of medicine in a protected environment in a manner that would hopefully lead to increased sensitivity to the psychosocial aspects of patient care (Rosenberg, 1973). Finally, devising mechanisms to identify those who are vulnerable to stress early on and providing timely assistance without stigma are essential steps in a successful program of prevention. It is only through such comprehensive efforts that the problem of physician impairment can be effectively tackled.

Erica R. Serlin, Ph.D
Formerly Assistant Director Student Affairs Office and
Instructor, Department of Psychiatry
Medical College of Ohio at Toledo
Toledo, Ohio

References

American Medical Association Council on Mental Health. The sick physician (impairment by psychiatric disorders, including alcoholism and drug dependence). *The Journal of the American Medical Association*, February 1973, 223(6), 684–687.

Cody, J. The M.D.eity: Some personality vulnerabilities of physicians. *The Journal of the Kansas Medical Society*, November 1978, 79(11), 605–607.

Coombs, R. H. *Mastering medicine: Professional socialization in medical school*. New York: The Free Press, 1978.

Coste, C. Resident impairment: The risky business of becoming a doctor. *The New Physician*, April 1978, 27(4), 28–31.

Derdeyn, A. P. The physician's work and marriage. *International Journal of Psychiatry in Medicine*, 1978–1979, 9(3 & 4), 297–306.

Funkenstein, D. H. The learning and personal development of medical students and the recent changes in universities and medical schools. *Journal of Medical Education*, 1968, 43, 883–897.

Herrington, R. E. The impaired physician—recognition, diagnosis, and treatment. *Wisconsin Medical Journal*, March 1979, 78, 21–23.

Rosenberg, C. L. Doctor rehabilitation. It is working. *Medical Economics*, November 26, 1979, 56, 114–122.

Rosenberg, P. Student's concerns during their first year in medical school. *Journal of Medical Education*, 1973, 48, 336–338.

Vaillant, G. E., Sobowale, N. C., & McArthur, C. Some psychologic vulnerabilities of physicians. *The New England Journal of Medicine*, August 1972, 287(8), 372–375.

Suggested Readings

American College of Legal Medicine Panel of Experts. What can you do about an impaired physician? *Legal Aspects of Medical Practice*, April 1980, 8(4), 40–49.

Duffy, J. J., & Litin, E. M. *The emotional health of physicians*. Springfield, Ill.: Charles C. Thomas, 1967.

Impaired physicians: Medicine bites the bullet. *Medical World News*, July 24, 1978.

Nadelson, C. C. & Notman, M. T. Adaptation to stress in physicians. In E. C. Shapiro & L. M. Lowenstein (Eds.), *Becoming a physician: Development of values and attitudes in medicine*. Cambridge, Mass.: Ballinger, 1979.

9 / Rite of Passage
Introducing Residents to Organized Medicine

Background
After 10 years in private family practice and working with a local Academy of Family Physicians, I relocated and became a director of a family practice residency. The program was active and contained a full complement of 18 residents. The residents were developing satisfactorily in their skills, attitudes, and medical knowledge in the field of family medicine.

One area of deficit which I encountered was that the previous director had not encouraged the residents to participate in membership or in attendance of the American Academy of Family Physicians organization at either the local, state, or national levels.

The Incident
After being settled in the residency for three months, I made contact with the local Academy of Family Physicians. I encouraged four of our second- and third-year residents to attend the quarterly academy meeting. The meeting was held in a private dining room of a local restaurant with approximately 30 practicing family physicians present, most of them over age 50. During the gathering the bar was busy and practicing doctor talked with practicing doctor, ignoring the residents and me. Finally, I felt the need to break the ice and introduced the residents and myself to several of the family physicians.

The conversation varied in topics such as: there are already too many doctors; the stock market; being ripped off by the welfare system; and the statement that I was no longer one of them since I had left private practice. I felt very uncomfortable and could see that my residents were being turned off by the whole scene.

After a fine dinner, the business meeting consisted of two portions: the election of delegates to the state convention, and a local political matter. After a heated discussion, the delegates were elected with the most vocal person being included. The physician sitting next to me remarked that the elected delegate was drunk, as usual. The big item which consumed most of the evening was a discussion concerning one of the elder family physicians who had been arrested for writing controlled drug prescriptions without examining patients. He was present to explain his case and felt that he had been "entrapped." A narcotics agent, posing as a patient, had received a prescription without proper examination. The physician was a long-time member of the group, and the group felt that they should help to defend him. This was listed as another example of government interference.

It was a long and quiet ride home with the residents after the meeting. The next day I gathered them to discuss the situation. The residents were disappointed, disillusioned, and angry. I had a difficult time listening since I shared some of the same feelings. They felt that if this was organized medicine, they didn't want any part of it. I tried to explain that not all groups have similar goals and leadership. I told them it was necessary that they become involved to change the course of organized medicine's goals and methods and to achieve a better professional and health care system.

Discussion

I am uncertain, at this time, what to do. Should I continue to encourage the residents to attend these business meetings? Should I try to become more involved with the officers of the local academy? Should I encourage the officers to become more involved in the residency? How do I deal with my own frustration?

Commentary

I cannot help but wonder whether the program director's predecessor had no interest in organized medicine or whether he was more aware of the local situation and chose to avoid it. Whatever the reason, the residents had had no exposure to organized medicine. Their new director's intent to correct this, starting with the local academy, was commendable. The fact that the experience was far from adequate and very frustrating to all concerned is apparent.

The new director had been settled into this large program only three months. Obviously, he had been consumed by this process and had little opportunity to meet the community physicians. To select a quarterly academy meeting to meet 30 of them for the first time and bring along several of the residents as well was a mistake. What transpired was not unusual and the reactions not unpredictable. None of the community physicians identified with the teaching program. They felt that the director had given up private practice and "was no longer one of them." A classical town–gown evening ensued. If the program director had been forewarned and had prepared his residents for this, I have no doubt that their degree of maturity would have enabled them to cope with the situation. When the incident concluded, his comments to the residents were excellent. However, it was most unfortunate that this had to be their introduction to organized medicine.

A very necessary part of family residents' training is their introduction to the medical community. This process has to begin at the local level where, hopefully, a number of the community physicians can become involved in the teaching program and learn to relate to the residents. Officers of the local academy should be invited to join the residency program committee and along with the other academy members be encouraged to serve as preceptors. In time this should lead to the invitation to participate in quarterly local academy meetings and to join the state and national academies as well.

Residents must learn that they are not expected to agree with or endorse all that transpires in organized medicine. If they disagree they should work from within for change. All of us should share the desire together "to achieve a better profession and health care system." The input from the doctors in training is just as essential, if not more so, as that from those of us over 50.

The program director in this incident answers his own questions very well. He should continue to encourage his residents to participate. He should become more involved with the officers of the local academy and should encourage them to become more involved in the residency. If he is successful in this, his frustration will take care of itself.

B. Leslie Huffman, Jr., M.D.
Clinical Professor, Family Practice
Medical College of Ohio at Toledo
Toledo, Ohio

Commentary

We are dealing in this situation with the attitudes of a newly hired residency director, the attitudes of his four residents, and the attitudes of the family physicians gathered for their quarterly meeting.

The emotional response evoked by the group of family physicians can partly be explained by their background. First of all, the age of the group averaged in the 50s. This group was raised in the years of the Depression, when jobs were at a premium. The attitude was one of long hard work with faithfulness to one job and job satisfaction from the fruits of long hours of work. Threat to job security or job satisfaction is posed by the welfare system inequities, the increase in the numbers of doctors, which creates competition, the decline of the stock market, and the perceived intrusion of a residency director who is no longer one of them. Older in years, this group feels they must stick together against government intrusion, and this may explain why the group defends a seemingly guilty physician. Jealousy may also arise from the perceived fact that younger physicians are better trained and better equipped to handle patient encounters.

In defense of the family physician group, do they not have the right to "let their hair down" after a tension-filled day at the office or hospital? There are not many occasions where a family physician, or for that matter any physician, can socialize without being constantly reminded of his or her position. Second, is it fair for the resident to make a judgment purely on one encounter? Most of the time a resident will interact with a physician in an office or hospital setting and judgment perhaps should be withheld until a profile of many encounters is established. Third, the residency director is credulous in his thinking by agreeing with the residents in his own mind without further investigation.

The residents' average age is 25 and their backgrounds differ substantially from the family physician group. The residents were raised during the era when jobs were plentiful, and their families had better lives, more money, and greater opportunity. The antiestablishment attitude was strong during the training years, leading to a different value system from the 50-plus age group. The 50-plus age group who were down on hippies, pill poppers, pot smokers, and antiestablishment attitudes now find themselves to be inebriated and faced with the possibility of one member breaking the law. More important, they are under careful scrutiny by a younger group with high ideals, perhaps too high expectations. The younger group exhibits self-righteousness and judges on one encounter.

The residency director, presumably about 35–40 years old, is in part molded by the World War II era where angry Americans fought to win at all costs. People raised in this era are highly conscientious and proud. I perceive the residency director as a highly conscientious, model family physician who spent 10 years in private practice, practicing good medicine. He enjoys education, keeps up with continuing medical education, and has devoted extra time to his academy to help promote its ideals. As a model family physician he attempts to rid the residency of any deficiencies by introducing his residents to the academy. In his present encounter he is bucking the label of the "new guy on the block." He no longer is viewed as one of the group. Perhaps he is no longer able to experience the frustrations of a private practice.

The residency director should begin by contacting the officers of the local academy and developing a program which can be presented at one of the quarterly meetings. The family physicians have so much to offer the residents by way of practice experience. The feeling of insecurity and misunderstanding as a teacher or educator must be dealt with, and satisfaction from teaching must be incorporated. Teachers themselves can be students who learn from the people they teach. The residency director should encourage several of the family physicians to precept in the model unit or take residents into their individual offices.

Contact should be made with the state academy of family physicians where the views of other family physicians as well as residents are heard. Perhaps an officer from the state academy who is well-respected can visit the residency program with a key resident who can explain academy functions and leadership potential.

In conclusion, the attitudes of all three groups, the family physicians, the residency director, and the residents, are understandable and predictable by the nature of their backgrounds and experience. Lack of communication promotes fear, distrust, and inappropriate decisions. Good communication engenders faith, pride, and good decision making.

Gary E. Ruoff, M.D.
Private Practice
Westside Family Medical Center
Kalamazoo, Michigan

II / The Professionals

Many of the critical incidents and issues encountered in family practice do not arise from the vagaries of the profession or the patient so much as from the actions, reactions, and interactions of health care professionals. This section, "The Professionals," is a collection of cases and commentaries selected to illustrate such incidents and issues. They are instructive not only because of what they reveal about the professionals involved, that is, ourselves, but what is learned about the pressures and conflicts that engender problematic, dysfunctional, and disruptive interrelationships among health care professionals.

Conversely, many of the pressures and conflicts inherent to professional training and practice are created by differences in the personal and/or professional philosophy, perspective, bias, knowledge, experience, and approach of the practitioners of various disciplines or specialties attempting to solve the same problem(s) or care for the same patient(s), especially when such differences are not mutually appreciated and respected. These differences are accentuated and the conflicts and pressures compounded by an erroneous assumption commonly held by many health professionals; that someone must be at fault—often ourselves—if a given problem, incident, or issue cannot be brought to satisfactory resolution, even though there may be no known good or easy solution. The strong emotions, most often negative, associated with such fault-finding tend to remain, unresolved, with the parties involved for a long time, perpetuating the differences, conflicts, and pressures and, in turn, giving rise to new incidents.

The cases in this section provide a wide range of such incidents. However, the solutions, approaches, and philosophies offered by the commentators also demonstrate the differences between professionals, even within the same discipline or specialty. The incidents fall within two general categories—those occurring between physicians and those involving physicians and nonphysician professionals. One of the physicians is always a family practitioner or resident; the nonphysician is most commonly a nurse, but hospital administrators and other health professionals are also involved. What is common to the case presentations in this section is that all of the incidents and issues revolve around patient care and the relative, often disparate, roles of the practitioners in that care.

This should not surprise the reader familiar with the sincere dedication of most health professionals to the patient's welfare and their enthusiasm for their own special perspective and approach to that care. For this reason, incidents and issues between the professionals will probably continue. And that is probably as it should be. However, when patient care becomes a mask and/or rationalization for personal, professional, and/or specialty self-interest, professional relationships become dysfunctional and patient care is compromised. The resultant incidents and issues then are truly critical.

Distinctions between patient welfare and professional welfare are not always easily discerned or maintained. The reader should be alert to this dilemma both while reading this section and in his or her own professional life. If the cases and commentaries in this section are helpful in accomplishing this end, its goal is realized.

The Editors

10 / In Loco Parentis

Medical Decision Making for the Incompetent Patient

Background

The incident occurred as I left my solo family practice to accept a salaried position in another state, but the problem had its origins many years before. The patient was a 46-year-old male who had severe mental retardation, present since birth. He lived with a married brother and sister-in-law and was capable of performing only a few simple household chores. His caretakers were both employed and the patient spent most days alone at home watching television, answering neither door nor telephone.

I was the family physician for the patient, his brother, and sister-in-law as well as for a number of extended family members living in the local community. There was a family history of polycystic kidney disease, and I had diagnosed this disorder when the patient was age 35. Hyptension had developed soon after, and during the past 10 years progressive blood pressure elevation had been accompanied by marked kidney enlargement and increasing renal failure. Despite medical therapy, the patient's blood pressure averaged 170/110 mm Hg. Renal function had deteriorated rapidly over the past year with glomerular filtration rate declining to 8 ml per minute.

I called a meeting of all family members and discussed the problem. This was an open and mutually supportive group who had aided the caretaking couple for two decades. There was concern not only for the welfare of the patient, but for the needs and feelings of all family members. We discussed

77

the various options available: hemodialysis, renal transplantation, or continued medical management now likely to culminate in the patient's death before too many more months passed.

The family examined their resources and the appropriate use of hemodialysis and renal transplantation. They also discussed what was "right" for the patient and for the brother and sister-in-law who had spent many years in caring for this individual. Finally, they examined their feelings about the decisions that must be made. After much discussion, the family unanimously agreed that the patient should be managed by current methods of medical therapy and that the options of hemodialysis and renal transplantation (which they perceived as "extreme measures to prolong life") should not be explored further.

The Incident

Deterioration of the patient's condition coincided with my planned departure from the practice. The care of most patients in the practice was transferred to a new physician in town who did not know either the patient or the family. When the case in question was discussed with the physician during transfer of the practice, he responded emphatically: "I don't care what the family says. This patient needs a hospital work-up and then probably hemodialysis until we can arrange a kidney transplant. The family does not have the right to make the decision that they have made, and it would be medically wrong to allow this patient to die when his life can be prolonged by available medical means. The first time I see this patient, I am going to insist that he be admitted to the hospital for evaluation."

The topic of this patient continued to arise during discussions of the practice transfer. In introducing the new physician to patients, I was able to introduce him to several members of the family. Eventually, we reached the tenuous compromise that he would see the patient, review the problem with the family, and withhold making recommendations until he had become personally acquainted with the case. I left the practice feeling some concern for the continuing care of this patient and family.

I have now been away from the practice and community for more than a year, but the mail brings the local weekly newspaper. I have seen no notice of this patient's death in the obituary column. I sometimes wonder whether this individual has received hemodialysis or even renal transplantation. Or is he still alive under medical therapy?

Discussion

This critical incident raises a constellation of issues concerning family responsibility, the appropriate use of resources, and philosophical differences between physicians. Did the family have the right to decide that the retarded family member with renal failure should not be considered for hemodialysis or renal transplantation? In this instance, was my first obligation to the family or to the patient? Did I have the right to agree to abide by the family's decision? In fact, was I correct in calling a family conference in which this decision was almost certain to occur?

And what about the appropriate use of resources? Are hemodialysis and renal transplantation really "extreme measures"? Can we as physicians make the value judgment that it is more appropriate to use scarce resources for employable, mentally competent individuals in preference to those who are unemployable or even retarded? Can I, as the family physician, make this decision? Is it better left to a panel that is less informed concerning the family problem—thus also more objective?

What about my philosophic differences with the physician assuming care of the case? Does he have any obligation to follow the course I had charted? Was I right in encouraging him to follow my plan of management? Was our compromise—that he would see the patient a few times before making a firm decision—really acceptable? When I learned that there was a difference of philosophy, should I have referred this patient and family to another physician for continuing care?

Commentary

The issues raised by this case history are commonly faced by family physicians, that is, the ethics of medical decision making when the patient is mentally incompetent. Patients may have congenital mental retardation, as in this instance, or mental incompetence may result from head trauma, mental illness, or organic brain disease. Each situation has unique clinical aspects, but the ethical, legal, and procedural principles form a recurring pattern.

Did the family have the right to decide that the patient should not have hemodialysis or be considered for renal transplant? Assuming they were reasonably intelligent, ethical people (and the description gives no hint that they were not), the family, once properly informed about the medical issues, has the prime authority and responsibility for decision making on behalf of the patient. Physicians often feel that because medicine has a mode of treatment to offer, all patients with a particular disease or condition should automatically have the therapy which is medically popular at the time. Further, they feel that if the patient or family declines, there is something inherently wrong with their judgment. The issue becomes somewhat more complicated when family members must make decisions on behalf of a mentally incompetent patient. However, the same principle applies.

The basic issues in this case involve the role and responsibilities of the physician versus the role and responsibilities of the patient and/or family in medical decision making. There are essentially two philosophical positions, each with variations, which physicians and patients and/or families can take.

These two positions are seldom explicitly stated but tend to lurk beneath the conscious level and subtly but powerfully influence both intellectual processes and emotional responses.

One position conceptualizes the individual and the family as the prime locus of decision-making authority in personal and family matters such as health care, economics, education, and religious beliefs. Experts in fields such as medicine, banking, education, and theology are viewed as resources which can be called upon and utilized as the individual and family see fit. The locus of control in the family is given primary authority and responsibility, and their decisions should be modified or overridden by outside people and organizations only when self-injurious acts or activities which injure others have occurred or are likely to occur (e.g., child abuse).

The second philosophical position assumes that socially recognized experts (such as physicians or educators) outside the individual and family are wiser than the person or family concerned and that the advice of the outside experts should be routinely followed. Carried to its logical conclusion, the second position implies that every individual and family should have a panel of expert advisors that makes all major decisions on their behalf. The physician makes the medical decisions, the educational advisor tells where and how to be educated.

Philosophically, our society is committed to the first position, that is, maximizing the opportunity for freedom of thought and decision making by individuals and family units. Practically, because some do not handle this responsibility very well and because of the increasing complexity of medical care, outside agencies such as legislative bodies and the courts are asked to intervene. Thus, laws and court decisions increasingly attempt to write rules and principles which define and protect the rights of the individual and clarify the responsibilities of the physician.

Returning to the discussion case, the first physician, who provided information to the family and helped them work through the medical and emotional issues involved, was playing the role of *advisor to* but *not decision maker for the family*. The second physician was operating on the "expert panel" concept and initially was inclined to preempt the family's right and responsibility under the philosophical system in which we live.

Both physicians have not only the right but the responsibility to abide by the family's decision. Their long-time family physician did exactly what every ethical physician should do in circumstances such as this: consult the family, inform them of the medical options available, make a personal recommendation if knowledge and experience suggests that a particular course of action has some clear advantages, then back off and give the family emotional freedom to reach their own decision. If there is a court-appointed guardian with full guardianship authority, that person has the ultimate legal authority to make decisions in the patient's behalf. If close relatives other than the guardian are available, the guardian should be encouraged to consult with them. The physician should be willing to participate in the consultation process. It is generally wiser to allow enough time to try for consensus among close family members if one is not dealing with an emergency situation. Consensus can ordinarily be reached more quickly if there are no major economic issues, for example, inheritance, large medical bills, which will especially benefit or harm one family member in relationship to others as a consequence of choosing among available courses of action.

The question of appropriate use of resources is a complex one and raises issues of "quality of life" as well of the presence or absence of key physiologic functions and the criteria by which limited health care dollars and resources will be distributed. These are ethical more than medical decisions. Ethics are reflections of one's philosophy of life and concept of man's place and purpose in the universe. Once again, two opposite philosophical positions can be stated and, depending upon which one favors, the ethics of the decision in question are derived.

The first portion is that physiologic life, in any form, is always to be valued above physiologic death and that no price is too great to pay for the preservation of physiologic life. This position supports the continuation of life support systems, if necessary, even though the brain or other major organs have ceased their normal function and cannot reasonably be expected to recover. The second position holds that in order to be valuable, human life must have perceptible meaning or the future possibility of meaning to the individual. Further, the current or potential existence of meaning can be detected or predicted with a reasonable assurance by others (trained professionals, family, etc.). As used here, *meaning* refers to the ability to carry out certain critical functions which differentiate human beings from other forms of life, that is, the ability to receive and respond to communication from other human beings and the ability to learn and periodically perform at least some autonomous functions requiring voluntary intellectual control. Meaning also implies observable evidence of the ability to exercise the human will and experience positive human emotions (joy, satisfaction, pleasure). This position further holds that when these conditions are not met, death can be merciful, not only to the person concerned but secondarily to ones who love the patient as well. Death is as natural as life and should not be unduly deterred by medical means when death may, in fact, be preferable to life.

Advocates of the second position would hold that preserving limited physiologic function where personality has a low probability of ever experiencing "meaning" is cruel and degrading to human life. One is then preserving a "thing," not a person, and it is the person, not the body, that gives worth to human life.

Our own personal feelings about death strongly influence where we fit on the continuum between these two opposing viewpoints since we unconsciously tend to project our personal feelings into decisions about patients. Those who fear death most (usually younger physicians) will gravitate to the "preservation of physiologic-life-at-any-cost" point of view. Those who feel that dehumanized life or a life of constant agony and deterioration is worse than death adhere to the "death can be merciful" view. When one integrates life philosophy with philosophy about the use of limited medical resources, ethical decisions can be reached that one can personally live with, even though others may differ.

In the case under discussion, the retarded man meets some of the criteria outlined above for "meaningful life." He was able to stay in the house alone during the day, watch TV, and perform a few other basic functions. The case history does not describe what his apparent emotional life was nor how frequently, if ever, he gave evidence of experiencing positive emotions. Did he have enough brain substance to have an emotional life or was his primarily a vegetative existence? Who was in the best position to make this inference? The family! They had known him since childhood. They obviously loved him because he was given a home rather than being placed in an institution. The brother and sister-in-law, in particular, were in a position to see whether there were day-to-day fluctuations in affect and infer better than anyone else whether life had significance for the patient. Given their obvious concern and sense of responsibility for his well-being, even though they may be tiring of their task, they could be trusted more than other fallible humans to make a sound decision in his behalf.

Employability is only one gross measure of whether to invoke costly technological medical procedures in behalf of a patient. The basic issue is whether extended life would be meaningful to the patient and to those who love him. The decision was "right" for his family because they reached it in the proper manner. If, for their own reasons, they had decided in favor of dialysis or transplantation, it would have been the family physician's responsibility to help them obtain a nephrologist's opinion, but not necessarily to insist that the family's wishes be carried out if the nephrologist disagreed. Whatever the outcome, the family physician's continuing role is that of providing emotional support, liaison with other care-givers, and information to help the family work their way through the many dilemmas to be faced.

If the new physician did not appear to be mature enough to fulfill a supportive role, the original physician could have suggested an alternative source of medical care by someone more philosophically attuned to the family's viewpoint and decision.

There often are no clear right and wrong ethics in a decision *per se*. The *process by which decisions are reached* is the clearest reflection of the ethical qualities of a medical decision. It is in this process that the physician has the opportunity to demonstrate the highest ideals of the profession.

Joseph W. Hess, M.D.
Professor and Chairman
Department of Family Medicine
Wayne State University
Detroit, Michigan

Commentary

In this case the family physician encountered situations which caused him to reflect on his obligations to the patient and his family as well as his relationship to another physician. The patient, a severely retarded 46-year-old male with a ten-year history of kidney disease, is, for all practical purposes, not able to assume the role of an autonomous person capable of exercising free and informed consent. It appears appropriate for the physician to assume that the family members will be the surrogate decision makers for this patient. The patient's good is inextricably related to the family context. Although we do not know what the wishes of the patient might be, it is not stated nor implied that the patient's desires are contrary to the views expressed by the family.

A family conference was desirable for several reasons. In the first place, the critical nature of the situation was openly and explicitly discussed. The treatment options were directly confronted by the decision makers. The patient's welfare was perceived in the context of his relationship to others rather than as an isolated medical problem. In the family conference, responsibility for the treatment decision was acknowledged and shared. The family doctor could have proceeded according to his best judgment without a full discussion of alternatives or consequences. The family might have played a passive role by placing the full burden on the physician by saying something such as "Whatever you say, doctor; you know best."

My impression is that this family physician would not have been comfortable with assuming full responsibility for deciding the course of treatment. The relationship between doctor and family was one of mutual trust and respect. This is in contrast to the apparent paternalism expressed by the new physician in town, who intended to insist on his own treatment plan in spite of the family's wishes. The new physician expected to be the primary decision maker.

Some might propose that an objective third party should be selected to speak for a patient who is unable to understand or speak for himself. It is possible that family members may be unable to distinguish the patient's welfare from their own needs. Occasionally, legal proceedings have been initiated to "protect" an incompetent patient from the bias of health care providers or family members. An example of the former is the case of Joseph Saikewicz, a 67-year-old resident of a state institution, who was so profoundly retarded he was unable to communicate verbally, and there were no family members available and willing to represent his interests. Chemotherapy treatment was considered for Mr. Saikewicz after he was diagnosed as suffering from acute myeloblastic monocytic leukemia in 1976. Referral to the probate court resulted in the appointment of a guardian *ad litem,* a decision not to treat, and finally an appeal to a higher court (Curran, 1978).

The case of Earle Spring, a 78-year-old incompetent patient suffering from kidney disease, was publicized in 1980. The family's decision to discontinue renal dialysis, although approved by the court, faced further legal challenges after several nurses objected to ending the regular dialysis treatments. In both the Saikewicz and Spring cases, a legal resolution of the treatment decision was not reached before the death of the patient. The resort to an objective third party through the courts is seldom a desirable and practical solution for determining the welfare of patients unable to exercise their own judgment (Relman, 1978).

Respect for the dignity of each patient and affirmation of life are important values. The incompetent patient has a right to be valued as a person independent of his or her contribution to society. The justification for the choice of treatment ought not be influenced by the patient's capability to be a self-sufficient and productive member of society.

In the case of this 46-year-old male suffering from acute renal disease, the appropriateness of treatment is relative to his medical, mental, and social condition. If it is presumed that his disease will result in death before many months, the consequences of the alternatives must be considered. The success of hemodialysis will be affected by the patient's mental and emotional ability to cope with the trauma of repeated treatments. It may be difficult to argue that hemodialysis will be correlated positively with an improvement in the quality of life. I would view hemodialysis, as well as a renal transplant, as an extraordinary means to sustain life. Extraordinary means are permissible, but not required. The use of extraordinary means requires that the probable benefits to the patient justify the burdens the patient will suffer. The obligation to minimize physical suffering through palliative treatment is greater than that of simply maximizing the length of life. Postponing impending death may be inflicting harm rather than doing good in some instances.

The relationship between physician and patient is an implied contract (Veatch, 1972). Ideally, there is a mutuality of consent and cooperation. For children and mentally incompetent adults, the patient may be represented by a proxy. Although the values of the physician and the patient may differ, each should respect the autonomy of the other insofar as possible. If the physician declines to enter into a contract with a patient or subsequently withdraws his or her services to the person, the relationship is not that of a physician–patient agreement.

When the family physician leaves his practice in the community, he severs his contractual bond with former patients. In the case under consideration, he transferred his practice to the new physician. If the new physician and the family jointly agree to enter into the physician–patient relationship, they will implicitly form a new contract. Should the family choose not to accept the new physician and his expertise, the 46-year-old retarded man will not be his patient. If the family rejects the approach of the new physician, they are, of course, free to seek another physician.

The willingness of the family physician to share his understanding of the patient and his family with the new physician was beneficial to all parties. Once he has left his practice, however, he is obligated to respect the autonomy of the new physician in managing his patients. He cannot interfere unless he feels compelled as a matter of conscience to protest an immoral or illegal act. The departing physician fulfilled his obligation by discussing the situation with the new physician.

The use of extraordinary life-sustaining procedures has implications for the allocation of scarce resources. Dialysis treatments would not impose an unreasonable burden on the family since the payment by the government is provided under amendments to the Social Security Act for cases of this type. Hopefully, the physician will not encourage initiating dialysis unless there is a reasonable prospect of benefit to the patient in comparison with the other therapeutic alternatives available. While it may be tempting to do everything possible for a patient, such a course is not always justified medically, socially, and financially. Eventually we may have to decide whether we want to invest an increasingly large proportion of our national resources in medical care. The marginal benefits of pursuing extraordinary or heroic measures for some might limit what may be done for others whose long-term health status is affected significantly by less-than-heroic means. The increasing role of third-party payments for health services in an economy of finite resources challenges us to make a thoughtful reevaluation of our ideals.

Ronald E. Benson, Ph.D.
Executive Director, Georgia Endowment for the Humanities
Emory University
Atlanta, Georgia

Professor of Philosophy
Ohio Northern University
Ada, Ohio

References

Curran, W. J. The Saikewicz decision. *New England Journal of Medicine,* 1978, *298*, 499–500.

Relman, A. S. The Saikewicz decision: Judges as physicians. *New England Journal of Medicine,* 1978, *298*, 508–509.

Veatch, R. M. Models for ethical medicine in a revolutionary age. *Hastings Center Report,* 1972, *2*, 5–7.

Suggested Readings

Annas, G. J. The incompetent's right to die: The case of Joseph Saikewicz. *Hastings Center Report,* 1978, *8*, 21–23.

Crane, D. *The sanctity of social life: Physicians' treatment of critically ill patients.* New York: Russell Sage Foundation, 1975.

Fox, R. C., & Swazey, J. P. *The courage to fail: A social view of organ transplants and dialysis.* Chicago: University of Chicago Press, 1974.

11 / "Where's My Doctor?"

The Physician Off Duty: Coverage,
Communication, and Conflict

Background

A level-II family practice resident was on call for the Family Health Center for the upcoming weekend and had the responsibility of taking care of the obstetrical patients of another level-II resident who was on vacation. The patient involved was a 24-year-old primiparous female whose expected date of confinement (EDC) was January 22, 1980. She had requested delivery at our Alternative Birth Center where the birthing process is allowed to take place in a home-like environment within the hospital. There is very little conventional medical intervention, and both parents participate in the experience. Both parents attended childbirth preparation classes and enthusiastically anticipated the new addition to their family.

The prenatal course was uneventful. One month prior to the EDC, ultrasound was consistent with 36.5-week gestational age and vertex presentation. Progress was satisfactory to the fortieth week of gestation. At this time it was mutually decided to induce labor. At this point, however, the primary resident physician left on vacation and the patient was referred to a resident colleague for further care. The family now understood that delivery could no longer take place in the Alternative Birth Center because induction was anticipated.

The Incident

Subsequent to admission to Labor and Delivery and adequate explanation of the induction process, the patient and her husband became very anxious. They demanded that the vacationing resident physician be summoned. Obligingly, the resident involved telephoned his vacationing colleague at home to discuss the situation with him and ask his assistance.

The telephone was answered by the spouse of the vacationing resident. The caller identified himself and asked to speak with her husband. The wife's reply led the caller to believe that the vacationing resident had gone out of town. This information was conveyed to the family, who seemed to understand the situation. Approximately five minutes later the vacationing resident appeared in the delivery suite, much to the amazement of the patient, the stand-in resident, and the delivery room attendants. He explained to the patient his vacation status, family responsibilities, and plans to leave town; then he left. When asked about the situation by the stand-in resident, the vacationing resident replied, "I did not tell my wife that."

The incident was immediately reported to the residency director by the stand-in resident, who was angry and embarrassed. He felt that the "lie" told by the spouse of the vacationing resident had produced the following effects: (1) significantly impaired the physician–patient relationship; (2) aroused his concern as to the effect this incident would have on his future relationship with the vacationing resident; and (3) most of all, compromised the quality of care delivered to the family concerned. The initial reaction of the program director to the incident was one of anger. But, upon reflection, he decided that the essential issue was conflict between personal and professional needs. The stand-in resident continued to complain to his other colleagues.

Discussion of the incident between the stand-in resident, program director, and social work consultant focused not on whether the vacationing resident had an obligation to deliver the patient, but on the stand-in resident's humiliation when his friend showed up, the loss of confidence in the stand-in resident on the part of the patient, the resident's anger at being lied to (as he perceived it) by the wife of his colleague, the vacationing resident's responsibility for his wife's presumed "lie," and what might appropriately be done to redress the issue. The stand-in resident was also concerned about losing his friendship with the vacationing resident. The suggestion was made that the vacationing resident may have been promising patients more than he could realistically deliver and that his personal-professional style and these patient expectations might represent a continuing potential for conflict between personal and professional needs.

An initial conference with the vacationing resident upon his return revealed the following: (1) His appearance at the hospital was purely coincidental. Actually, he had stopped off at the hospital on his way out of town to collect his paycheck. On entering the hospital lobby, he met the father of the family involved, who informed him of the day's events. The resident then went to make a courtesy call on the patient, whereupon he encountered his colleague. (2) The entire incident has resulted in a strained relationship between the two residents concerned as well as their respective families.

The situation remains unresolved and the mechanism by which resolution could be accomplished still evades us. Separate conferences with each resident yielded different perceptions of the facts, significance, and implications of the incident. The resident who filled in for the vacationing resident is still convinced that he was lied to by his colleague's wife and that since the incident compromised the quality of care to the family concerned, the vacationing resident should be disciplined. The residents were each encouraged, individually, to discuss the matter between themselves.

Discussion

This incident raised many issues in the author's mind. How does one deal with retrospective situations when it is so difficult to ascertain the facts? To what extent do an expectant mother and her spouse have the right to expect her physician to be present for the delivery? What are the limitations on such rights? What responsibilities do physicians on vacation or otherwise off duty, with previous arrangements for practice coverage, have toward their patients or the colleagues covering that practice? How does a spouse resolve the dilemma between protecting the physician's privacy when off duty, and, at the same time, maintaining appropriate communications with the physician's patients and colleagues?

Problems that bring physicians before boards of censors or other peer review organizations are many and varied, but often relate to personal problems, communication problems, marital problems, and interphysician relationships. This incident stands out as a warning to the author that a resident physician is at risk for developing many of these problems with professional ramifications.

The major problem for residency faculty, however, seems to be the management of these situations without invading the resident's right to privacy. What is the role of the program director in such a situation? Where does administration and teaching end and therapy begin? Can physicians be held accountable for their spouses' actions? Does a spouse have the option of protecting the physician's right to privacy and relaxation when off duty? In the residency setting, how can a spouse's attitude toward and/or conflict about the physician's professional life be detected? Most of all, however, what support services for residents can be designed to adequately deal with incidents such as the one described?

Commentary

Although there are several important issues raised in this critical incident, they can be grouped into two general categories. The first deals with patient and physician rights and responsibilities when a physician is off duty. The second centers around communication skills and needs. It contains several important aspects: the necessity of developing and maintaining channels of communication between colleagues and between the physician and patient; what can happen when open communication does not occur; the importance of communication between house officers and program directors; and a spouse's responsibility in this communication.

Let us first consider the issues surrounding patient and physician rights and responsibilities. Once a doctor assumes responsibility for a patient's care, he has that responsibility whether he is on or off duty. If unavailable, he must delegate that responsibility. The patient then has the right to receive appropriate care when the physician services are required. After that, the issues become more complex because the physician also has the right of privacy and of off-duty time. When, and by whom, is it decided that a patient's condition requires immediate care by a particular physician? In the past this posed fewer problems since practicing physicians were always on call and interns were literally "interned" in a hospital for 365 days. In this system, the doctor's privacy and rights to off-duty hours were sacrificed. Societal values have changed considerably, and it is doubtful that there will be a significant swing back to the old ways. Instead, new arrangements in health care have developed: group practice, partnership, and coverage schedules which have created more humane hours for house officers and practicing physicians alike. These changes provide continuous care for patients at all times and allow the physician to reserve some time for extra-professional activities. In general, these systems work, as evidenced by the growth of such practice arrangements and the falling number of solo practice physicians.

However, gray areas remain. Even though the vacationing resident in this incident had legally discharged his responsibility in making certain that his patient was receiving competent health care, did he have the moral and ethical obligation to render that care himself? After all, she was his patient. Was her care compromised by his absence? Although this poses a dilemma, it also raises a question of judgment and flexibility, two characteristics a physician should have. The off-duty physician has to weigh several factors: Is the patient's need for his personal services real or perceived? Will his presence make a difference? What are the physician's off-duty commitments—is he catching a plane for China or staying in town?—and can he improve the situation by staying on duty for a short period of time and taking leave when the situation is under control? His patient's well-being comes first as he gathers the data. Obviously, the decision that is reached depends on individual interpretation, and this should be rooted in the knowledge that a clear understanding of responsibilities has been established before the episode occurs. Many family practice training programs notify their patients in writing when the patients are enrolled that they will be cared for by a certain physician or, in his absence, a member of that physician's team. What is meant by being off duty should also be spelled out clearly for patients and house staff.

Given that any such situation can be satisfactorily handled only on the spot, the reported incident indicates that the off-duty resident failed to take time to assess the situation and to provide a smooth transition. It may take a few minutes or many hours to relieve a patient's anxiety. However, to an even greater extent, the covering resident failed in his duties. It appears that he conveyed to the patient his anger and resentment of the off-duty resident. He also continued to pursue the matter in a belligerent fashion. Although he professed to be concerned about losing his friendship with the off-duty resident, he went to the program director, continued to insist on disciplinary action, refused to accept the off-duty resident's claim that his wife was uninformed about his whereabouts, and insisted that he was lied to by his colleague's wife. Such hostility seems out of proportion to the incident and suggests to me—and undoubtedly to the program director as well—that these two house officers harbored smoldering, unresolved conflicts that were brought out by the reported episode.

This entire critical incident, then, really centers around poor communication and lack of empathy. This incident could have been defused if the off-duty resident had informed the covering resident of his travel plans, if the off-duty resident had adequately communicated to his patient his plans and his concerns for her care, and if he could have reassured her that she was in good hands. He also should have communicated with his wife. In any good relationship, a spouse becomes a part of the health care team. It is important, then, that spouses recognize the role they play and be prepared to handle it. They must accept the physician's obligation to his patients.

How, then, are these values and communication skills to be taught? To a large degree, they seem to be to be inborn, but they can be improved. Some family practice programs spend a week or even a month in intensive orientation of incoming residents before the residency begins. Parts of this orientation are conducted with the spouses. At the completion of the orientation, house officers select a colleague(s) with whom they will share rotations for the next three years. These selections are hopefully made, in part, on the basis of easy, open communication between these partners, obviously lacking in the two physicians described.

Since issues that came up in this critical incident (and elsewhere in this book) occur commonly, it might be helpful to discuss such issues in advance and even have role-playing sessions with open discussions. Similarly, after these incidents happen—and of course they will continue to occur—the program director should use such episodes to further the learning, understanding, and communication skills of the house officers. In the present incident a meeting between the program director and both residents should be held. The purpose should not be to affix blame, but together to analyze the situation to see why it arose, what would have constituted more appropriate responses, and how it managed to engender such hostility. The incident should be turned into a learning and growing experience.

Rooted in this seemingly insignificant incident is the basic question of what comprises standard professional behavior. Regardless of the profession, one must maintain an effective, positive relation with one's colleagues. One must also be responsible, whether it is to one's patients or clients. And most important, perhaps, is the professional's personal integrity and self-respect.

Lewis B. Morrow, M.D.
Professor of Medicine
Associate Dean of Clinical Affairs
Medical College of Ohio at Toledo
Toledo, Ohio

Commentary

The incident described indeed raises many issues regarding physician–patient and physician–physician interactions. The primary problem appears to be one of communication between the two physicians involved, which then coincidentally involves patient care and interfamily conflicts.

In analyzing the situation as presented, there is a question as to the level of comfort of the covering resident in assuming the care of the pregnant patient and being a substitute at delivery for the vacationing resident. One of the mechanisms which can be used to avert some of the emotional and communication problems which occurred in this incident is for any physician to assure and to be responsible for informing a covering physician of all aspects of the case, medical and nonmedical, thereby ascertaining the feelings and attitudes of the covering physician prior to the transfer of responsibility. This includes discussing any potential medical complications or unusual conditions which might make an impact upon the care of the patient, any previous understandings and commitments which the physician has made with the patient regarding medical care, any special or unusual circumstances that are anticipated, and the results of discussions with the patient and family regarding their feelings about the patient's condition and its care. It is also helpful if the physician who is leaving communicates his wishes to be informed of any complications or to be contacted during his time off. The anger engendered by the reappearance of the vacationing resident could not have produced such a subsequent strain between the two individuals had they, at that time, been able to continue a dialogue which had been started much earlier by sitting down and discussing their feelings, reasons for the reappearance at the hospital, and plans for dealing with the patient. The covering resident would have determined the reason for his anger and then been able to deal with and discuss that reason with the vacationing resident. It appears that as the "hurt" progressively assimilated into the emotions of the two residents, their ability to deal with it and each other in an effective manner decreased with time.

It is difficult to conceive that patient care would have been compromised had communication channels been opened early and maintained. The lack of communication continued, however, as evidenced by the loss of confidence and strained relationships which evolved between the two individuals. At the point that this became a significant impairment to the ability of the two residents to function together, it was the program director's responsibility to gather information and to encourage the two individuals to mutually solve the problem. Failing this, it was the residency director's responsibility to sit down with the two individuals in a nonthreatening atmosphere and request that they share with each other their feelings regarding the situation and their perception of the occurrences, and to jointly negotiate a resolution of the problem. In doing so, the residency director could have employed some of the techniques of negotiation he had acquired in dealing with administrative problems as well as his behavioral science skills in the area of crisis intervention. It is important that the two individuals involved be helped to recognize the strain which the incident had placed upon the relationship and the importance of learning how to deal with such potential problems in the future. The continued disharmony produced by a lack of cooperative and problem-solving communication between the two individuals could have made a major impact upon the functioning of the entire class of second-year residents and the residency as a whole. A program director's responsibility includes the appropriate role modeling of ways of solving interprofessional conflicts. Should those conflicts proceed to a point where one or both individuals are unable to deal effectively with their anger and/or perceived humiliation to the extent that their performance becomes impaired, appropriate therapy should be recommended.

The use of a sponsor system, team system, and/or an "open door" policy to the full-time faculty is important in affirming to the resident that the program is indeed concerned and committed to helping residents investigate and resolve conflicts. By providing individuals who can serve as support persons within the residency program, individual residents can be made to feel that they can bring problems to such individuals in a nonjudgmental atmosphere.

It is my feeling that support systems can be designed to adequately deal with such incidents as this one if faculty and ancillary personnel look upon their responsibility as, not merely the teaching of organic knowledge, but also role modeling the function of the family physician as counselor and friend. Some programs have appropriately used a sponsor system by assigning an attending faculty member who can function outside the residency setting as a resource person to the individual resident in resolving conflicts involving both the residency and personal issues. Another approach is the team system, in which residents can be grouped so as to provide feedback and support for each other in dealing with stresses during the training years. It is important in any of these strategies that a variety of communication styles be utilized. As this process takes place, each resident can learn various ways of communicating with peers, family members, and other significant people in his life. Among the important aspects of support systems are the use of an open feedback mechanism and a nonjudgmental attitude in dealing with the various conflicts and incidents which do occur. Specific sessions regarding conflict resolution can be utilized to discuss how other individuals approach problems, avoid incidents, and resolve such incidents once they have occurred.

Another issue raised by this incident is the legitimate expectations of patients for the presence of their personal physician and the limits of those expectations. Again, these revolve around the physician's communication of his role and responsibilities to each individual patient and the contract to which the physician has verbally and/or nonverbally committed himself. It is important at the time the physician communicates to the patient his availability that he also discuss the patient's expectations of the physician. Patient expectations of physicians are many times colored by their previous experiences, their parental tapes, and their security needs at the time of a specific illness. The physician should discuss with the patient that the need for priorities within his life will result in there being times when he will be unavailable. It is incumbent upon the physician to inform the patient that arrangements are made for practice coverage and that pertinent aspects of care will be delegated to a covering physician.

The final issue raised by this incident regards the physician–spouse interaction. In the residency setting, spouses' attitudes do have impact upon professional life and performance of the resident. Again, this relates to a question of communication between the two individuals, their ground rules, and their preferences for handling different situations. One of the responsibilities of the marriage bond is for the two individuals to communicate with each other regarding the responsibilities and attitudes of each and to negotiate the important aspects of the relationship. This can be solved in a number of ways, but it is important that there be agreement between the physician and the spouse in defining their relationship. It is also important that the division of responsibility be communicated to others who will be involved with the physician, including his partners, peers, and other people who have frequent communication with the physician himself.

The characteristic stresses of residency training have been documented in several studies. It is apparent that all involved in the described incident— resident substitute, vacationing resident, their families, the program director, and other faculty—were under stress. Because of this stress, they focused on their own personal needs and secondary issues rather than on the primary issue of the care of the patient and family. This incident reaffirms the need for psychosocial support systems in residency training programs. Such systems might include: (1) support groups that meet together regularly, with or without a leader, for the purpose of sharing problems, feelings, and support; (2) part-time residency and/or shortening the number of residency hours per day or days per week, but lengthening the duration of residency training; (3) formal "gripe sessions," defined as scheduled times when residents can bring complaints about the program before the director; and (4) seminars and/or speakers, both dealing with emotion-laden medical issues and the stresses of being a physician. Seigel and Donnelly conclude that, "primary prevention of later personal difficulties should be recognized as a goal of medical education. Within a medical training program, attention to the emotional needs of each trainee is likely to have both short-term and long-term benefits for the intern, her/his family, her/his patients, and the medical profession" (1978, p. 914).

David L. Hoff, M.D.
Professor of Family Medicine
Akron City Hospital
Northeastern Ohio Universities College of Medicine
Akron, Ohio

Reference

Siegel, B., & Donnelly, J. C. Enriching personal and professional development: The experience of a support group for interns. *Journal of Medical Education*, 1978, 53, 908–914.

12 / To Heal or Steal?
The Doctor–Patient–Doctor Relationship

Background

As a third-year resident in family medicine, I have lived in a Midwestern city for one-and-one-half years. The home which my family and I rent is approximately five minutes away from the major teaching hospital and the family practice center with which I am associated. Our landlord and his family are very congenial and amiable people, and a very good relationship has been formed between our families. It has not been infrequent for me to treat numerous members of the landlord's family when acute, relatively nonserious problems, such as lacerations, have occurred because the family did not have a primary care physician and did not frequent any doctor for continuous medical care.

The Incident

One evening my landlord approached me and stated that his 78-year-old father had been quite short of breath for approximately one week. He stated that his father's personal physician had seen him two or three days prior to our conversation, but the medical regime prescribed had not been very effective in the landlord's opinion. He was quite concerned that his father's condition was becoming worse. As a result, he asked me if I would be able to examine his dad in my office in the near future. I accepted this challenge and advised my landlord to bring his father to my office the following morning. After a thorough examination, a diagnosis of congestive heart failure was made. The patient was placed on a diuretic, responded appropriately, and was feeling much better within two or three days. I saw the patient three times in the following eight days. From the first visit, it was apparent that the shortness of breath was not just an acute, simple problem, but that this symptom related to some long-standing pathology. It became readily apparent that I had placed myself in a difficult position by inviting him to come to my office for treatment, not really being his primary care physician and, especially, since the patient had seen his own physician approximately five days prior to his seeing me.

Discussion

Several dilemmas arose. First, it was difficult to explain to the patient that I, or the other physician, would have to see him on a continuing basis. I explained to the patient that he really had to decide whether he wished to continue being followed by his original physician or transfer his care to me. The problem was compounded by the fact that he had been going to his primary care physician for many years and really had no complaints about his care in the past. Another dilemma occurred to me. If the patient chose to transfer his care to me, it would be rather awkward for me to explain to his original physician how I had become involved in the case. The patient took three or four weeks to decide. After consultation with other family members, he chose to transfer his care to me. However, I did not feel very comfortable in this situation. I certainly felt that by agreeing to see a patient who already had a physician, perhaps I had overstepped my bounds without considering the consequences that might result.

Commentary

The physician in this incident faces the transformation of a casual Band-aid service into a formal doctor–patient relationship. Defining the boundaries of the doctor–patient relationship is crucial for any decision he makes regarding this transformation. The resident must decide whether to refer the landlord's father back to his primary physician, arrange consultation with another, or accept the request personally.

What is the doctor–patient relationship and what expectations govern the conduct of this relationship? Doctor and patient meet for the purpose of restoring or confirming the presence of the patient's health. To understand the meaning of this relationship, one must examine the socially expected roles of both physician and patient. Further, one must examine the factors enhancing the therapeutic outcome of this relationship.

The physician enters the relationship as a professional helper invested by society with the authority to perform diagnostic and therapeutic maneuvers that define and alleviate the disease process. Further, he is sanctioned by society to grant an individual the rights of the "sick role" (Bowden & Burstein, 1974). The "sick role" in our culture has five aspects: (1) the assumption that the person is incapacitated through no fault of his own; (2) the right to have the need for care by another person met; (3) exemption from usual social obligations; (4) recognition that the person is ill with a desire to get well and return to social functioning; and (5) the expectation that the ill person will cooperate with his physician and adhere to a treatment regimen.

In order to fulfill his role, the physician is allowed privileges uncommon in other relationships. He has the right to explore the private and confidential areas of the patient's psychosociobiological makeup as well as examine the patient's body. In return, the physician is expected to demonstrate a high level of technical competence and to treat his patients scientifically, based on objective criteria rather than personal feelings. He is expected to limit his treatment to areas of his technical competence and maintain objectivity by refraining from personal involvement with the patient. Last, he is expected to put the welfare of the patient before his own in the practice of medicine (Leigh & Reiser, 1980).

The patient enters the relationship at his discretion (often encouraged by family or friends) and does so for a variety of reasons. He may seek relief from pain. He may be worried about the implication of a symptom. He may have a variety of somatic complaints that reflect problems in living. Covertly, he may seek refuge in the sick role in order to obtain compensation or privileges of the sick. His employer may require certification of his health status in order to perform a job. Last, he may come for a routine examination and the subsequent reassurance of health (McWhinney, 1972). Regardless of the reason, the patient controls the formation of the relationship by deciding when to see the physician and which physician to see.

After establishing contact with a physician, the patient will elect to maintain the relationship or shop for another. The decision depends upon the "feel" of the relationship. If the physician fulfills the societal role previously described and demonstrates empathy by listening to the patient and tempering the therapy to the patient's needs, a positive feeling will ensue. With this feeling comes a sense of trust and, subsequently, the belief that the relationship is beneficial. The patient's belief in the relationship has a healing impact of its own which is unrelated to the specific effects of the doctor's treatment (Benson, 1979). Consequently, the therapeutic outcome of a fully developed relationship exceeds the obvious benefits derived from a drug or surgery alone. For this reason, development and support of the doctor–patient relationship remains vitally important to the practice of medicine.

With respect to the incident several pertinent questions arise from the previous discussion:

1.   What motivating factors underlie this visit?

2. How strong is the patient's relationship to his primary physician?
3. What effect will the decision to treat have on the patient's relationship to his primary physician?
4. In view of his friendship with the landlord's family, can the resident fulfill the socially expected role of doctor?

Attempting to resolve these questions may facilitate the final decision of which physician should be involved in a doctor–patient relationship with this man.

Why has the landlord's father come for help? Had he notified his physician that he wasn't responding to treatment? Was he dissatisfied with his physician, or was he being encouraged by the family to see another doctor? The answers to these questions are important in deciding whether to support the primary physician or whether a new relationship is needed. If the patient is comfortable with his primary physician despite his lack of improvement, then referral for follow-up would be indicated. However, if he is uncomfortable about his failure to improve, he must be questioned about his wish for another opinion. If he wishes to maintain the relationship with his primary physician, a second opinion should be arranged through his primary physician. If he does not wish to return, a second opinion could be arranged independently. Failure to ask these questions and to decide accordingly may lead to an intrusion on the care and trust previously developed. This is important if the patient desires to return to his primary physician for ongoing follow-up. Only when the patient has clearly decided that no further contact is desired should the resident initiate a new relationship.

Whether or not the resident should assume personal care depends upon his ability to fulfill the role of physician. Does his relationship to the family affect the diagnostic or therapeutic outcome of this man? Can he remain objective or nonjudgmental? Would the patient be hesitant to share information that would be more readily shared with a physician having no association with the family? If the physician's objectivity is skewed or he is unable to maintain emotional neutrality, he may have difficulties developing a beneficial doctor–patient relationship and should refer to another physician.

The resident's concern about ongoing follow-up would, I believe, be resolved with the development of trust and empathy. In the context of the relationship described, it would be important to probe and understand the implications of this disease on the patient's life. Additionally, it would be important to understand the patient's perception of the health care system as derived from his prior contact and comments from friends or family. The process of active listening itself may facilitate this patient's agreement for ongoing medical care as well as ameliorate the impact of this problem.

This physician faced a difficult problem common to doctors at all levels of training: the request for help from family and friends. The problem that arose in this incident stemmed from his passive acceptance of the doctor–patient relationship without prior examination of its implications. Had he examined the implications, his decision may have been the same but his delivery of care would have been shaped with a clear idea of his capabilities and his limitations.

Brian Schmitt, M.D.
Assistant Professor of Family Medicine
Medical College of Ohio at Toledo
Toledo, Ohio

References

Benson, H. *The mind/body effect*. New York: Simon and Schuster, 1979.

Bowden, C., & Burstein, A. *Psychosocial basis of medical practice: An introduction to human behavior*. Baltimore: Williams & Wilkins, 1974.

Leigh, H., & Reiser, M. *The patient: Biological, psychological, and social dimensions of medical practice*. New York: Plenum, 1980.

McWhinney, I. "Beyond diagnosis." *New England Journal of Medicine*, 1972, 287, 384–387.

Commentary

It must be emphasized that the physician involved in the incident is a family practice resident. As such, his response to the request to see another physician's patient must be considered somewhat differently than would a similar request of a privately practicing physician. To a physician outside a training program, the incident presented would probably be no dilemma because such situations are a rather routine part of practice. It would be appropriate for a private physician to simply suggest that the patient may be best served by returning to his personal physician promptly, but if the patient should so choose, the private physician would be happy to see him for either a second opinion or potential continuing care.

As a third-year resident, the physician in the case described two dilemmas which developed because he saw the patient of another physician. First, the resident felt difficulty in explaining to the patient that a physician would have to see the patient on a continuing basis and that the patient would have to decide from whom he wished to receive his care. I believe that this presents less of a dilemma than an opportunity to provide the patient with some education and some insight into the philosophy of family practice. Patients do require long-term care for chronic problems. Also, patients do have to decide from whom they shall receive their care at the same time avoiding excessive "doctor shopping." Both the tenets of good patient education and the philosophy of family practice, which include continuing care for the patient, would indicate that the responsibility for these choices lies with the patient and the patient's family and that the patient and family can be best served by providing competent and compassionate continuing care by a personal family physician.

The second dilemma discussed revolved around the need to explain to the original physician how the resident had become involved in the case. It is not stated whether or not the resident knew the original physician, nor is it stated whether or not the original physician was associated with the residency in any way. If the resident had no prior or continuing relationship with the original physician, I suggest that no explanation is necessary. A routine office-to-office request for the medical records is all that is in order. If the original practicing physician is a friend or is associated with the residency in a substantial way, I suggest that an informal "over coffee" comment to the original physician is all that is necessary. That may be simply a brief discussion initiated by a question, "Say, do you remember . . ." Unless there are extenuating circumstances not apparent in the case described, I do not believe the resident overstepped his bounds and that he can rest assured that this type of situation is a very common and real-life situation which will occur frequently in future practice.

Perhaps the dilemmas presented by the resident could have been avoided through handling the situation a bit differently right from the start. The resident's landlord did not have a primary care physician and did not see any physician for continuous medical care. As the resident physician developed a relationship with the landlord and his family, perhaps the resident could have encouraged the family to seek their medical care in a more appropriate fashion. Although we all are called upon to render some facets of episodic care to our neighbors occasionally, it may have been appropriate to encourage the entire family to see the resident or some other personal physician on a coordinated and continuous basis. Perhaps an opportunity to promote good family practice was missed.

The resident's anxiety regarding the provision of care to the elderly gentleman with shortness of breath could perhaps have been alleviated by proceeding a bit differently from the outset. If the elderly gentleman's condition was actually worsening despite treatment prescribed by the original physician, perhaps the patient could have been encouraged to contact the original physician immediately to describe the situation and ask for a prompt reappraisal. If the patient did not wish to do this, or if the original physician was unable to see the patient right away, then perhaps the resident could have telephoned the original physician to briefly advise him of the patient and ask if he had any suggestions or recommendations based upon the original care rendered. If such advice had been offered, or if a telephone call had been made to the original physician at the outset, the evolution of the situation into a continuing relationship should not have provoked considerable anxiety.

The medical profession has but few guidelines regarding the provision of care to the patient of another physician. The International Code of Medical

Ethics as adopted by the World Medical Association in 1949 states that "a doctor must not entice patients from his colleagues" (1949). It does not appear as though the resident physician enticed the patient away from another physician, but rather responded to a quite legitimate request for a second opinion and then for subsequent transfer of care from another physician to himself.

The Opinions and Reports of the Judicial Council, prepared and approved by the Judicial Council of the American Medical Association in 1977, speak to the point that patients have free choice in their selection of a physician. "Free choice of physicians is the right of any individual. The individual may select and change at will the physicians who serve him. . . . The freedom of the individual to select his preferred system of medical care and free competition among physicians and alternative systems of medical care are prerequisites of ethical practice and optimal medical care" (AMA, 1977).

The American Academy of Family Physicians has also indicated that the patient's right to free choice of physician is preeminent. The AAFP stated in 1959 that "The AAFP strongly upholds free choice of physician as a concept to be considered as a fundamental principle—incontrovertible, unalterable, and essential to good medical care" (AAFP, 1980).

The dilemmas posed by the third-year family practice resident are certainly more complex than the truism that patients have a right to choose their own physicians. Perhaps because it is only in recent years that physicians in training have had true doctor–patient relationships that there are apparently no guidelines which can be followed regarding the interactions between a resident physician who acts in the capacity of a personal physician and the private practicing physicians in a community. Perhaps it is good that there is a relative absence of such guidelines because the doctor-to-doctor and doctor-to-patient relationship can then develop in a manner appropriate to the unique setting in which each resident and residency exists.

Daniel J. Ostergaard, M.D.
Director
Duluth Family Practice Residency
Duluth, Minnesota

References

American Academy of Family Physicians. *Academy policy on key health issues, ready reference guide, 1979–1980*. Kansas City, Missouri: Author, 1980.

American Medical Association Judicial Council. *Opinions and reports of The Judicial Council*. Chicago: Author, 1977.

World Medical Association. *International code of medical ethics*. New York: Author, 1949.

13 / Practice What You Teach
The Practice Competence of Teaching Faculty

Background

The meeting was not due to start for another 20 minutes, yet a few participants had begun to gather. The cold, wintry weather and recent snowstorm had induced the knowledgeable to get an early start. There were also a few who had traveled from other time zones and were uncertain of their alertness. I had met only a few of these physician-educators previously, yet I had heard of most of them. Their experience and prestige were overwhelming. So I stood alone and surveyed the room. Groups of three or four clustered about the windows and along the table. Others strolled in and out of the room.

The Incident

It must have been at least five minutes later that I summoned enough courage to amble about. This made me less conspicuously alone and also afforded me the opportunity to catch a few pearls from these sage educators. Suddenly, I was aghast at the scene in front of me. In the midst of this tranquil setting, a man, whom I did not recognize, was lying on the floor. He was receiving CPR from several others I did know. After several seconds of staring, I became aware of the inappropriate, meager efforts to resuscitate the heavy-set individual, whose skin was ashen. I quickly walked away. I joined a group standing at some distance, but with a view of this staggering scene. They were reviewing the onset of the person's discomfort and his concern for his postprandial heartburn. I was told who he was. This sent me reeling toward the hall. I knew him.

As I reached the door, I turned and went back to the man's side. At close range the efforts of the resuscitators seemed even more ridiculous. The actions were inexperienced and uncoordinated. Just weeks earlier I had completed the American Heart Association CPR course for physicians. I was now taking the instructor course. I had complained that it was ridiculous to require all the residents and faculty to take the Basic Life Support Course. After all, they used CPR all the time in the emergency room and at the bedside. How could these physicians not have the same basic knowledge or experience? What were they doing? They were not a team, but a disorganized duo.

I stepped forward and began as first assistant. Then I took over. When the nurse and ambulance crew arrived, they helped with the ventilation and started an IV. Despite all the appropriate procedures, we got minimal response. Then a few short spontaneous breaths and pulses gave me hope. But we were running low on available medications. I sensed the size of the crowd in the room growing. I was being watched. We needed some more medications! They were not here, but in a hospital. We got ready to depart.

In the ambulance, the previous triumphs disappeared. Terminal vomiting revealed the air in the victim's stomach from inadequately performed ventilation prior to the insertion of the endotracheal tube. We continued our efforts in the rolling ambulance, as well as the emergency room, but there was no more hope. I was sunken. Worse yet, when I returned to the meeting, it had not yet begun and only a few participants seemed to be at all shaken. They were the victim's closest colleagues. I was consoled by those few, but after that the matter was dropped.

Discussion

My biggest problem was to restrain myself from seeking out those involved and lecturing them on coordinated two-person CPR. How could they be involved in patient care, with residents or students, without knowing effective CPR? What could I do to help them? How could I prevent this in other faculty? Why had I not stepped in sooner? How would they now react to my having taken over for them? How would they react to my hesitancy? Several years have passed. Can I still take a stand?

Commentary

Society's expectations of physicians include the ability to perform in an emergency situation. The most important medical emergency, claiming 1,000 lives per day in the United States, is sudden cardiac death (SCD), as exemplified by the case in point. This physician's initial distress was that these prestigious physician-educators were unable to perform a basic life-saving procedure. In other words, they fell short of his expectations as physicians.

We tend to ascribe omniscience to our mentors, but how often in a teaching situation, where the contact with each patient is likely to be episodic, is overall basic quality care ignored in the interest of an esoteric diagnosis? As the physician implies, medical students and house staff expect not only that their teachers can understand the physiology and etiology of cardiac arrest, but also that they can demonstrate the psychomotor skills necessary to treat it. Examined in a broader perspective, our medical educators may have credibility only if they are proficient in the practical skills as well as the spectacular.

The physician's desire to immediately seek out the ineffective rescuers to lecture to them was best quelled at the time because the situation was so complicated by personal emotional factors. These emotions need to be recognized and dealt with since they can interfere with performance in an actual emergency situation. *Anger*, directed at himself and his colleagues, is apparent though not directly stated. *Fear* that he had not performed well and might be criticized for his initial hesitancy is an added dimension, as is *anxiety*, as he sensed the size of the crowd growing and knew he had to perform under the scrutiny of others. The seeming lack of concern of the victim's colleagues was more likely a defense mechanism, part of the protective shield physicians erect to help them in dealing with death. After all, our training has ingrained the concept that death is the doctor's enemy. In addition, the death of a patient, especially a colleague, reminds us of our own mortality. These psychological factors which attend resuscitative efforts are often ignored in training sessions, especially in physician CPR courses. Apparently, many think that the social and moral imperative that a physician is expected to save lives is enough to overcome the stresses involved in the actual situation. However, the emotional catharsis afforded by open discussion of these factors at the appropriate time is healthy for all physicians.

Although several years have passed since the physician experienced this situation, it still troubles him and he questions what he can do to prevent a similar situation with other faculty-physicians. The crisis was SCD and the first critical step in its management is immediate and effective CPR (Moss, 1980). This is the message he needs to deliver.

Since the introduction of closed chest massage for the treatment of cardiac arrest two decades ago (Kouwenhoven, Jude, & Knickerbocker, 1960), a standardized, systematic approach to CPR has been developed by the American Heart Association in conjunction with many other scientific organizations (Standards and Guidelines, 1980). In addition to the obvious and documented benefits of this form of medical therapy, Copley, Mantle, Rogers, Russell, and Rackley (1977); McIntyre, Parisi, Benefari, Goldberg, and Dalen (1978); and

McIntyre (1981) have shown that improper CPR techniques performed on a recording manikin correlate with pathophysiologic changes in man during resuscitation. Thus, insistence on the rigid standards of the American Heart Association program for CPR training can maximize chances for survival and minimize complications.

This nationally accepted program is being taught throughout the country, and an estimated 12 million citizens have had formal training that would enable them to effectively perform CPR (Dalen, Howe, Membrino, & McIntyre, 1980; Schwartz, Orkin, & Ellison, 1979). In an unannounced test held recently at the University of Colorado Medical Center, not one of the 45 interns and residents who responded to a simulated cardiac arrest situation passed (CPR exam, 1981). Should we not be as dismayed at these results as the physician in the preceding case history whose colleagues could not pass the test in a real-life situation? How can we require firemen, policemen, and many allied health personnel to be trained in CPR when we do not demand it of our own profession?

Although our own professional and personal integrity should be sufficient to demand our knowledge of basic life-saving skills, the present legal climate cannot be ignored. Failure of the responsible physician to initiate CPR or perform according to established standards may increase his risk of legal liability. In addition, many a lay person is now an informed critic and perhaps an "expert witness" to the physician's improper performance.

Physicians of all specialties should be competent in the basic life-support measures. The public looks to the medical profession for leadership and exemplary behavior in this regard. Since no other specialty in medicine can claim such diversity in terms of clinical or human experience as family practice, the communicative skills of the family physician could be effectively used to advance the cause of CPR training in the medical and lay communities. Following are recommendations and questions to aid in this goal:

Medical School:
1. Basic Cardiac Life Support (BCLS) training should begin in medical school: faculty needs to be convinced of this.
2. Advanced Cardiac Life Support (ACLS) should be taught before clinical rotations.
3. House staff and medical school faculty should be recertified each year.

Hospital Medical Staff:
1. Do you have recent certification in CPR?
2. Does your hospital offer CPR courses and yearly recertification as part of its CME program?
3. Does your hospital recommend or require CPR certification for reappointment to the medical staff?

4. Do your emergency room physicians have current training and certification in basic and advanced life support?

Office and Community:
1. Are your office personnel trained in CPR?
2. Do you recommend CPR training for spouses and families of patients at high risk for SCD?
3. Would you be willing to serve as advisor and/or instructor for organizations that are teaching CPR to lay and paramedical groups?

As physicians, we enjoy the privileges the title brings; it also brings accountability. Without scientific knowledge and skills, the compassionate wish of the physician to serve mankind's health means little.

Donna Ailport Woodson, M.D.
Private Family Practice
Clinical Associate Professor
Department of Family Medicine
Medical College of Ohio at Toledo
Toledo, Ohio

References

Copley, D. P., Mantle, J. A., Rogers, W. J., Russell, R. O., & Rackley, C. E. Improved outcome for prehospital cardiopulmonary collapse with resuscitation by bystanders. *Circulation,* 1977, *56,* 901–905.

CPR exam: House staffers all flunk. *Medical World News,* 1981, 22, 22–24.

Dalen, J. E., Howe, J. P., III, Membrino, G. E., McIntyre, K. Sounding board: CPR training for physicians. *New England Journal of Medicine,* 1980, *303,* 455–457.

Kouwenhoven, W. B., Jude, J. R., & Knickerbocker, G. G. Closed-chest cardiac massage. *Journal of the American Medical Association,* 1960, *173,* 1064–1067.

McIntyre, K. M. Basic curriculum: How to increase success of cardiopulmonary resuscitation. *Journal of Cardiovascular Medicine,* 1981, *6,* 531–541.

McIntyre, K. M., Parisi, A. F., Benefari, R., Goldberg, A. H., & Dalen, J. E. Pathophysiologic syndromes of cardiopulmonary resuscitation. *Archives of Internal Medicine,* 1978, *138,* 1130–1133.

Moss, A. J. Prediction and prevention of sudden cardiac death. *Annual Review of Medicine,* 1980, *31,* 1–14.

Schwartz, A. J., Orkin, F. K., Ellison, N. Anesthesiologists' training and knowledge of basic life support. *Anesthesiology,* 1979, *50,* 191–194.

Standards and guidelines for cardiopulmonary resuscitation (CPR) and emergency cardiac care (ECC). *Journal of the American Medical Association,* 1980, *244,* 453–509.

Commentary

My first reaction in reading this critical incident was that here was another Walter Mitty fantasy with the unfamed hero again distinguishing himself where those with worldwide recognition had failed. Upon completing my reading, I found that our hero was not successful, the patient died, and a variety of unresolved conflicts remained. This, unfortunately, made clear to me that this was a real-life incident without the happy ending of the Mitty stories.

I will discuss the issues raised here under the broad categories of clinical, educational, and ethical. The clinical issues relate to the value and use of CPR. The educational implications revolve around the larger question of teachers being capable of doing what they expect of their students. The ethical questions relate to individual and group responsibility.

Cardiopulmonary resuscitation (CPR) has led to the development of a new specialty (emergency medicine) and has involved the general public directly in the provision of acute medical care. In 1967, only physicians were believed capable of being trained to administer CPR. By 1974, the American Heart Association set a goal that one out of every four adults would become proficient in CPR. Out-of-hospital resuscitation, if administered within four to six minutes of collapse, will salvage 30 to 45 percent of victims to return to their prior state (Eisenberg, Bergner, & Hallstrom, 1979). If extended beyond this critical time, there is a rapid decline in survival rate.

CPR is a specific skill and like all skills requires constant practice to maintain true proficiency. In one study of trainees' retention of CPR techniques, most had lost their skills and knowledge when retested six months after training (Weaver, Ramirez, Dorfman, & Raizner, 1979). Physicians would be less likely to lose this skill because of a more complete understanding of the principles involved. Nevertheless, it is likely that those not often involved in CPR, for instance, physician-educators, would not be particularly proficient. A *JAMA* editorialist noted that emergency medical technicians (EMTs) expressed concern that physicians in their offices or at the scene of an emergency are not familiar with good standard resuscitative techniques and yet insist on maintaining control (Carden, 1979). This is true despite studies demonstrating that EMTs perform as well as recently trained physicians completely familiar with CPR.

CPR is an effective lifesaving skill. It is most effective when initiated immediately and when performed by those with frequent experience. In an acute emergency, the most proficient should administer CPR regardless of title or position.

The relevance of this critical incident to family practice education extends beyond the question of the competence in CPR of physician-educators. The essentials of training for family practice residents require knowledge and skill in the performance of CPR. If the general public, emergency medical technicians, residents, and practicing physicians are expected to be capable of performing CPR, certainly physician-educators should maintain this competency.

Extending this principle to other skills is not so clear. This is particularly so when physicians with various specialties are involved in residency training. Should the internist or pediatrician involved in family practice education develop skills in obstetrics? Should preceptors in the family health center be required to have competency in coronary care or intensive care units? By virtue of their limited role, it is understandable that these faculty members do not require this broad capability.

On the other hand, full-time family practice faculty are seen as role models for residents as well as being their teachers. If they do not possess the requisite skills, this may imply that the broad area claimed for family practice is really not practical. The oft-stated criticism that it is impossible to function adequately in so many medical fields may be confirmed if senior faculty are unable to do what they teach.

There are two responses to this concern. First, in a specialty that is so young, the truly expert practitioner-teacher is only now being trained and gaining experience. The newly trained family practice physician will have incorporated the knowledge and skills of his various mentors. He will then be able to apply these broad skills to practice and to teaching.

The other response is that no one is totally competent in all aspects of any specialty. Even in the narrowest specialties, further subdivision occurs. If this does happen in family practice, the subdivisions will remain broader and each subdivision will still be comprised of generalists.

We must conclude that in order to train the ideal family practitioner, we must have faculty as competent role models while recognizing that they cannot be expert in all of the areas of family medicine. Nevertheless, there are certain basic skills of competency expected of all. These would include not only the usually emphasized interpersonal skills but also the basic emergency skills of CPR. The emphasis in family practice is in training a physician who truly cares. The greatest demonstration of not caring is the lack of basic clinical competence.

The ethical issues raised by this incident fit into the general area of "responsibility." The core of the incident relates to the responsibility of the individual health care professional in the face of incompetence by his perceived superiors. This has broad clinical implications for residents and students, with faculty or preceptors, as well as nurses and technicians, and with attending or resident staff.

An even broader generalization can be made from this incident, relating it to individual responsibility in any field, including business and government, when one's superiors are perceived as committing grave errors. More than a single life is at risk when a general or a president makes an obvious error and his subordinates hesitate to intervene.

Responsibility then is a complex moral question, including one's judgment as to what is right and what degree of certainty exists in that judgment. It is not as simple as doing one's duty, which does not require a judgment.

The Nuremburg Trials, the My Lai incident, and the resignations in the justice department during the Watergate cover-up all establish the responsibility of individuals to disobey immoral orders. The active assumption of responsibility in the face of incompetence is less clear. In the *Caine* mutiny, those taking over the ship are not welcomed back as heroes.

It is likewise the responsibility of a nurse to refuse to administer a treatment she deems harmful to her patient. The fact that this is difficult and has a high potential for personal liability only emphasizes that responsibility is a complex moral issue. The decision to actively replace one's superiors who are performing inadequately requires a certainty of judgment beyond the refusal to carry out an order. Mutineers are considered guilty until proven innocent.

The decision involved in the critical incident described is even more difficult because of the urgency of the situation and because there is no constituted authority. Yet, in other ways, the responsible decision is more obvious. The author, recently trained in CPR, knows the proper technique and is certain that inadequate measures are in process. What prevents his immediate action is the awe of famous people and the disbelief that they could be in any way incompetent. Even many years later, as he relates this incident, the narrator remains concerned about how these luminaries view him. "How would they now react to my taking over for them? How would they react to my hesitancy?"

Responsibility requires judgment based on adequate information and reasonable certainty. It is usually difficult, but never more so than when questioning the competency of one's professional superiors.

The physician in this case now realizes that the responsible decision would have been to step in immediately and administer appropriate CPR. He feels guilty at his own hesitancy and disappointed in the response of the famous in his field. I share in his disbelief at the group's reaction to the sudden death of a colleague. If his recollection is accurate, their behavior should have been questioned at that time. Having failed to do so then, he would perform a valuable service to his profession by now surveying the CPR capabilities of physician-educators and sharing his results through a public forum. Having had this experience, it is his responsibility to do so. For all of us, it is our responsibility to maintain our clinical competence, to practice what we teach, and to come to an acceptance of the moral dilemma in accepting and giving up responsibility.

Joel H. Merenstein, M.D.
Director of Research
Family Practice Residency
St. Margaret Memorial Hospital
Pittsburgh, Pennsylvania

References

Carden, T. S. Emergency medical services—the bottom line. *Journal of the American Medical Association*, 1979, *241*(18), 1931–1932.

Eisenberg, M. S., Bergner, L., & Hallstrom, A. Cardiac resuscitation in the community: Importance of rapid provision and implications for program planning. *Journal of the American Medical Association*, 1979, *241*(8), 1905–1902.

Weaver, F. J., Ramirez, A. G., Dorfman, S. B., & Raizner, A. E. Trainees' retention of cardiopulmonary resuscitation. *Journal of the American Medical Association*, 1979, *241*(9), 901–903.

14 / "My First Reaction Was Disbelief"
Surgery without Medical Clearance

Background

The patient is a 62-year-old black woman with hypertension, chronic bronchial asthma, insulin-dependent diabetes, and moderate elevation of lipids.

Three years ago, the patient had a "cerebral hemorrhage" which left her hemiplegic with a contracted left hand. The patient is able to walk with the help of a tripod cane and is able to walk in her home without assistance since the "throw rugs" have been removed. The patient is cooperative. She keeps her appointments. She is not able to keep her blood sugar well controlled since she likes sweets. At times, she is "depressed" due to her condition.

The Incident

One night, around seven o'clock, I got a call at home from the recovery room nurse stating that my patient was in the recovery room with a blood pressure of 240/140, a tachycardia of 140, and hyperpnea of 28. The nurse informed me that the anesthesiologist was quite worried about the condition of the patient. I then inquired why the patient was in the recovery room and was told that our ENT man had removed a plaque from her palate and a lesion from her neck.

When the patient's blood pressure became elevated, the nurse called the ENT physician, who told her to find out from the family who her family doctor was and call him.

Discussion

My first reaction was disbelief. It seemed inconceivable to me that a patient who had so many medical problems would be operated upon without a "medical clearance." We have only two otolaryngologists in town, and they are in partnership. They, therefore, must receive all my consultations. When I asked for further details of the patient's care and condition from the nurse, the only thing I could find was that no insulin orders had been given. I also discovered that the ENT surgeon was making "evening" rounds in the hospital and asked the nurse to have him call me. When I had not received a call in two hours, I called the nurse back and found out that the ENT man had, indeed, written some orders for insulin coverage of glycosuria. An order for me to see the patient had not been written.

What now is my next approach? Should I confront the ENT man? Should I tell the patient that I do not feel that I want to take care of her since she is subjecting herself to "stress"?

The lesions on the patient proved to be benign. The patient was discharged home the next day. Fortunately, she has not suffered permanent sequelae from this incident.

Commentary

This incident raises various issues in medicine, including those that are asked at the conclusion of the incident. If I were confronted with the same issue, I would monitor the patient's progress by phone with the nurse and would not interfere with the patient's care unless the patient was in obvious danger. I would not confront the patient directly about this incident, but I would have an office employee call the patient to make sure that she was not having any problems during the recovery period. I would make certain the patient received increased patient education about the nature of her diseases and the relationship of those diseases to stress. It is quite obvious that this patient does not comprehend the seriousness of her medical illnesses.

In my experience, an incident like this, created by a physician in a very limited specialty, is not uncommon. Most physicians in such specialties do not read medical literature concerning general medical care, and as they become busier and busier in those narrow specialties, they involve themselves less and less with the overall health care of their patients. Part of the role of the family practice specialist is to recognize these situations as fact and protect the patient while, at the same time, trying to impress upon the limited specialist that the object of their care is a human being and not a disease.

The entire incident raises the issue of the organization of the medical staff at this hospital. This patient should be protected by the medical staff bylaws with a provision that no patient should undergo a general anesthetic without a complete history and physical upon that chart as required by the Joint Commission on Accreditation. It is the responsibility of the anesthesiologist to review that chart and to assure the patient's safety to undergo anesthesia. It is also the anesthesiologist's responsibility to monitor that patient's health status during the recovery period from the anesthetic. Therefore, the anesthesiologist has some responsibility in this incident. It is not entirely the error of the ENT man.

My approach to this problem would be based upon the past record of the otolaryngologist concerning similar incidents. If this were an isolated incident, I would gently suggest, on a one-to-one basis, that this was not the proper approach and that I would appreciate knowing when my patients were to be operated upon. If this instance was part of a pattern and happened on a regular basis, then I would definitely make an attempt to stop this poor quality of medical care. To do this, I would write the physician in question about my displeasure and would send a copy of such a letter to his partner, the chief of the medical staff, the hospital administrator, and the chairman of the board of trustees of the hospital. Over the years I have discovered that this approach may appear rather harsh, but it is also very effective when people in authority receive copies of such letters. The president of the board of trustees is the last resort, but he is responsible for the quality of care in the hospital.

Frank F. Snyder, M.D.
Clinical Associate Professor
Department of Family Practice
Medical College of Ohio at Toledo
Director, Family Practice Residency
The Toledo Hospital
Toledo, Ohio

Commentary

The "incident" described occurs all too often today and promises to increase in frequency, placing the patient in more and more jeopardy in the years ahead. The underlying causes are obvious, but first let us look at the incident and inject some calm and reason into the frustrated physician's description of the incident and the questions he asks.

What are the facts surrounding the incident? The patient had apparently contacted the ENT man directly concerning a problem with her palate and neck. He made the decision that an operation was indicated and preoperative evaluation by other physicians would not add to the safety of the patient. Whether or not his decision was correct, one cannot question his freedom to make that decision. He then performed the operation. The patient's recovery was complicated by hypertension, tachycardia, and hyperpnea. The nurse notified the ENT surgeon of the findings. He asked the nurse to identify the patient's family physician and "call him."

The communication process varies from hospital to hospital and community to community, but I interpret the ENT surgeon's communication to the nurse as a verbal order which she should have written in the chart. I also interpret the order as a call for consultation to the family physician. It then becomes the responsibility of the consultant to promptly respond and render consultation or decline, for whatever reason, in order that the consultation may be directed to another physician. "Disbelief" on the part of a physician has never been of assistance to a patient in need. The response we all wish and should expect from any consultant is a rapid assessment of our problem and a mature effort to quickly work through whatever administrative and other barriers exist in order to insure proper management of our illness or injury.

Now, let us consider the specific questions posed by the family physician:

"What now is my next approach?" Respond or decline promptly the next time you are consulted to aid a critically ill patient.

"Should I confront the ENT man?" No, a confrontation will not improve the communication between physicians or the care of the patient. If you, as a member of your medical society or hospital staff, feel he is incompetent or dishonest or unethical, then this matter should be dealt with by appropriate procedures. What would be helpful would be to invite the ENT man to sit down over a cup of coffee and then clarify how you wish to communicate so that future misunderstandings may be minimized.

"Should I tell the patient that I do not feel that I want to take care of her since she is subjecting herself to 'stress'?" Of course not! She needs you. Do what you can for her when she requests your assistance. Don't let her health care suffer because of the irritations and politics of practice. She is a 62-year-old woman with hypertension, chronic bronchial asthma, insulin-dependent diabetes, moderate elevation of lipids, and a plaque on her palate which I expect she thought was cancer.

Finally, the "root" of the matter or the underlying cause of the "incident": Ethically, morally, and traditionally every hospitalized patient has a right to expect a single physician to be in charge of his or her total care. Physicians and surgeons today threaten to make a mockery of this principle, perhaps the most important determinant of whether a patient survives the illness or injury.

Consultants are often essential, giving verbal advice to the physician in charge or writing recommendations for tests and treatment and suggestions regarding diagnosis. However, the dangerous practice of sharing responsibility for the patient has emerged in recent years with multiple physicians writing orders on the same patient. With this arrangement, no one physician bears the burden such that he provides the thought, planning, and action so vital to insure optimum care. This sharing of responsibility has progressed to the point where some surgeons no longer provide postoperative care and in time, like the ENT man, either refuse to manage postoperative problems or are incapable of doing so. Such a practice is unethical and condemned by the American College of Surgeons with the same disdain as fee-splitting. The practice of shared responsibility has also been contributed to by the primary care physician who is not content with the role of consultant in the postoperative care of his patient.

Let us all work together to stop this practice. During the course of a hospital stay it may be necessary and correct to transfer the patient from the care of one physician to another depending on what problem poses the major threat to the patient's life at a given time. At no time is it permissible to have several physicians all writing orders. Finally, we must all make an effort to improve our communication with one another for the benefit of our patients.

Neil R. Thomford, M.D.
Professor and Chairman
Department of Surgery
Medical College of Ohio
Toledo, Ohio

15 / "They Only Ask for Me When They Are in Trouble!"
The Dysfunctional Consultation

Background

The characters involved in this incident are:

1. An obstetrician—his relationship with the family practice residency program has been fraught with problems. There have been poor evaluations of him by the residents and some difficulties over previous referrals. Most of the residents prefer to work with one of his colleagues.
2. A patient who works in the hospital laboratory.
3. The patient's work colleagues.
4. The admitting resident.
5. The primary care physician, who is a new faculty member.
6. The hospital administrator.

The history is that of a female in her early 20s who presented with a history of severe menometrorrhagia. She had been treated for the preceding six weeks with hormone therapy by the primary physician. On the night of admission, she phoned the family practice resident on call to state that she was hemorrhaging and wished admission. The resident phoned the primary physician and the two of them agreed to admit the patient overnight and refer for dilatation and curettage (D&C) the following morning should the patient's history be confirmed by examination. At that time, the primary physician was a new faculty member and had not yet obtained D&C privileges at the hospital. The patient was admitted to the hospital and a consultation request made to the obstetrician. The following morning the primary physician went to see the patient around 10:00 A.M. Upon reviewing the nurses' notes, he discovered that the patient had not been bleeding at all overnight and that the hemoglobin and hematocrit were normal and stable, as they had been in the outpatient department. He asked whether the consultation had taken place and was informed that the obstetrician had refused to see the patient.

The Incident

The primary physician examined the patient and found minimal vaginal bleeding and a normal pelvic exam. Following the examination, the primary physician informed the patient that he had asked an obstetrician to review her case since the bleeding obviously was not being controlled by hormone therapy. The patient said, "Yes, I heard him in the passageway. He shouted at the nurses and said that he did not want to see that family practice patient. They only ask for me when they are in trouble." The patient stated that she was very upset and did not see why a member of the hospital staff should treat her like that. The primary physician promised that he would speak to the obstetrician, who was at that time the only member of the obstetrical and gynecological staff not out of town at a conference. He also informed the patient that since she was not bleeding heavily and her hemoglobin and hematocrit were stable, he did not feel that he could justify her remaining in the hospital. He would arrange for her to be seen by the obstetrician as an outpatient that afternoon, if possible. It so happened that he had referred the patient on an outpatient basis prior to the admission and the patient already had an appointment that afternoon.

During the following two hours the primary physician attempted to reach the obstetrician but was unable to talk to him personally. He was telephoned by the mother of the patient and by a member of the laboratory staff. Both inquired why a hemorrhaging patient was being sent out of the hospital without treatment. Questioning regarding whether this behavior constituted abandonment took place. Upon calling the obstetrician's office to confirm the outpatient appointment, the patient was informed that it had been canceled and that she would not be seen. Eventually, the primary physician tracked down the obstetrician, talked with him, and arranged for the patient to be seen that afternoon. The patient had an endometrial biopsy and was started on a hormonal regime with a view to D&C should this fail. A letter of complaint from the family was subsequently received by the hospital administrator.

Discussion

What was initially a simple request for help with a surgical D&C resulted in deterioration of relationships with the community obstetrician and the disruption of care to a difficult family.

Commentary

This critical incident presents issues which are not unique to obstetrics and gynecology. Rather, it reveals an image of the family physician as perceived by some patients and many colleagues in other specialties of medicine. There is also the problem of how to manage a patient whose clinical picture does not correlate with the history.

The initial problem in this case is for the family physician to convince the patient, her family, and her fellow employees in the laboratory that her medical problems are not as acute as she might have imagined and that time can safely be obtained by waiting. Certainly, a paraprofessional person would understand that if the hemoglobin and the hematocrit are stable, bleeding cannot be too great.

The clinical picture presented by this patient does not warrent acute care for a person in her 20s. If such a history of profuse bleeding occurred in an early menopausal or postmenopausal patient, the indications and the necessity for a D&C would be entirely different. The chances of this patient having a malignant process in the endometrium is extremely unlikely. At the worst, she might have a hyperplastic endometrium or an incomplete abortion.

An adept family physician should sit down with this patient and carefully explain to her the entire scope of her problems in terms that she would be able to understand. He should explain to her that it is many times harder to quantify the amount of menstrual bleeding and that what seems to be a great amount of blood to the patient is often not truly a pathologic amount when examined by the physician. Certainly, the patient should be started on oral iron. The choice of a medical D&C by hormonal therapy would not seem, to this writer, to be inappropriate.

The second, much more critical issue presented by this case is the relationship of family medicine to other specialties. It is unfortunately true that many specialists do not recognize the family physician as an equal colleague. All too often they feel that he is some type of a "second-class citizen" with limited abilities to cope with problems. These narrow-minded physicians fail to understand or perceive the high level of training that the family physician receives in both residency and postresidency continuing medical education. This writer would certainly disagree with the obstetrical consultant when he said that, "the family doctors only call when they are in trouble." Quite the contrary, family physicians often treat problems that they feel comfortable with, and when they have problems beyond their scope of training, they call for help. It is not only when they are in "trouble."

A frank, candid discussion with this obstetrician, once the emotional atmosphere has defervesced, would seem to be appropriate. This new faculty member in family medicine has to get along with the obstetrician as a fellow member of the medical community. Sitting down and having a discussion of the assets and liabilities of family medicine might help educate the person. My guess is that it will not. People of this particular emotional set are not often willing to listen to reason and I will predict that the family physicians in this particular community are going to continue to experience difficulty with this particular individual.

The fortunate thing about American medicine is that there is always a medical center within a reasonable distance, which can be consulted or to which the patient can be transferred. Such regional centers, even in the most sparsely populated areas of the Far West, are usually within easy travel time by the patient. When unilateral resistance is encountered as in this case, rather than debate or argue the issue, it might be much better to simply refer the patient to a regional center for another specialist's opinion.

All in all, one can appreciate how uncomfortable the family physician must have felt in this situation, and one can clearly understand why it has been described as a critical issue.

With the combination of careful explanation of the problem to the patient and her relatives, exploratory discussion of the situation with the antagonistic specialist, and, as a last resort, using referral to a regional center, some of the anxiety of such situations can be removed. However, there probably will always be strained relationships with such an antagonistic specialist.

John L. Duhring, M.D.
Professor and Chairman
Department of Obstetrics and Gynecology
Medical College of Ohio at Toledo
Toledo, Ohio

Commentary

I have been asked to consider the special problems that evolved as a result of a "simple request" for help with a surgical intervention. There is concern about the deterioration of the relationship with a community obstetrician, who was not well known to the physician requesting the consultation, and about the reasons for the disruption of care to a difficult family. Comments should also be made concerning the medical necessity for the consultation.

One of the most likely causes of menometrorrhagia in a female in her early 20s is dysfunctional uterine bleeding. Although there are various methods of treatment, hormone therapy, as outlined by several acceptable methods and regimens, usually resolves the problem in the purely dysfunctional bleeder (Alcheck, 1980; Brenner & Mishell, 1980). Assuming that the patient was, nevertheless, correctly treated prior to the consultation request, there are initial concerns that need be examined in the evolution of the events of this "simple" consultation.

The primary physician or the admitting family practice resident should have examined the patient immediately prior to admitting her. By so doing, both of these well-meaning physicians could have avoided what eventually proved to be a sensitive, troublesome incident. However, a consultation was requested before the patient was examined for this hospitalization (I suspect via orders given to a nurse). This particular sequence, as related in the "background" description is clearly in violation of the "Commandments of Consultation": "The request for consultation should be in writing; additionally, a verbal communication between the requesting physician and the consultant enhances the effectiveness of such a request. The consultation also should not be accomplished through a third party" (Burnside, 1973, p. 53).

It would have been more appropriate had the patient been seen by the obstetrician-gynecologist in his outpatient office before having to consider an elective surgical procedure in the hospital setting. It would have been far better to have allowed the consultant the freedom of management choice supported by the atmosphere of his own outpatient office. It is at this point that the whole issue of consultation versus referral rears its ugly head. There is at least some question in this particular incident as to whether the family physician should have referred, that is, transferred, the patient to the obstetrician-gynecologist in view of the degree of involvement which the primary physician anticipated he would have in this patient's care.

Consideration should be given to the demeanor and professionalism exhibited by the obstetrician-gynecologist in his relationship with the primary physician and the patient. Apparently, from the description in "The Incident," the consultant was quite busy because he was the only member of a group that was not away at a conference. This fact, however, was not the only possible reason for his inappropriate conduct; there had apparently been previous episodes which had caused residents in the hospital to prefer not to work with him. There are many reasons (none of them good) why a consultant would make the quoted statements about the referring physician, especially in the presence of his patient, inciting that patient, in an already tenuous situation, to suspect that her care might be compromised and not altogether the quality she had a right to expect. The factors are numerous and will not be discussed. Suffice it to say that this consultant's actions were entirely inappropriate and should not have occurred for any reason.

The reasons for the disruption of care to this difficult family are numerous and perhaps justified. This is a family who obviously has very definite ideas about the workings of a hospital and the doctor–patient relationships, and probably has some technical knowledge concerning the proposed surgical procedure. Unfortunately, families like the one described tend to be somewhat manipulative. That is quite obvious in the patient's ability to influence the admitting resident and, ultimately, the primary care physician to hospitalize her, an event which eventually led to the misunderstandings and difficulties which followed.

As with many patient–physician problems which result in varying degrees of misunderstandings and litigation, some blame can be directed toward each of the participants in the incident. What appeared to be a referral for a "simple surgical procedure" in this case was not really so uncomplicated, and the deterioration of the relationship between physicians was probably inevitable. It is clear that each participant contributed to the development of the problems which are described in the incident and to the eventual unpleasant experience and deterioration of relationships between the participants. Situations like this unfortunately still occur all too frequently.

John H. Coleman, M.D.
Director, Family Practice Residency Program
Mercy Hospital
Toledo, Ohio

References

Alcheck, A. Abnormal vaginal bleeding in adolescence. *Consultant*, 1980, 3(20), 103.

Brenner, P. F., & Mishell, D. R., Jr. Functional menstrual disorders. In H. Conn & R. Conn (Eds.), *Current diagnosis 6*. Philadelphia: Saunders, 1980.

Burnside, J. R. Commandments of consultants. *Hospital Physician*, 1973, 9, 53.

16 / The "Education" of a Consultant
Secondary Consultation: Rights and Responsibilities

Background
Dermatology was the last rotation for me in 1979. As a third-year resident, I spent that month dividing my time between my practice at the Family Practice Center and being an observer and assistant to the dermatologist associated with the medical college. My major objectives on this rotation were to see as many dermatologic problems as possible and to learn currently effective modes of therapy.

The Incident
Ninety-five percent of the patients who came to the dermatology clinic had been referred to the dermatologist by primary care physicians, both in and out of town, for dermatologic problems difficult to diagnose or resistant to therapy. In most instances, the patient's problem was managed to the satisfaction of both the patient and the referring doctor. On occasion, however, the patient or the patient's parents would ask the dermatologist about a problem that the patient had been experiencing that was unrelated either to dermatology or the reason for referral. For example, "What do you think about my headaches over the last two to three months?" In such cases, the dermatologist often chose a course of action that essentially involved advising the patient that he thought the problem should be evaluated by an appropriate secondary specialist, for instance, a neurologist, and that he would be very pleased to

make arrangements to have that patient seen in the indicated clinic at the medical college. Often, this could be arranged within the hour since the particular clinic needed was in session at that time. Frequently the patient or patients would leave the dermatology clinic, walk across the hall, and become a patient of the appropriate clinic involving the other complaints which they had. The fact that one "unit" chart was used by all of the clinics made the transition or referral even less complicated.

Discussion

I felt that this was contrary to good medical practice. In my opinion, the dermatologist really was stepping out of line by assessing problems (1) that were outside of his field of expertise and (2) for which the patient had not been referred. It seemed to me that it would have been more appropriate to return the patient to the primary care physician for evaluation of those nondermatological complaints or at least telephone the primary care physician for an opinion regarding referral to a "specialty" clinic.

This type of incident placed me in a dilemma. As a trainee in family practice, I disagreed with this policy. However, as a visitor to this service, I did not know whether it was my place to comment. Certainly, alienating the dermatologist at that time might have adverse consequences on the quality of the remainder of my rotation and the nature of our subsequent interaction. It was also an unfortunate possibility that if this specialist continued this particular practice, he might thereby inadvertently decrease the number of future referrals from primary care physicians who became annoyed at his referral of their patients without consultation. Yet I could readily perceive that the dermatologist was acting more out of ignorance of his role and prerogatives as a consultant than out of willful malice or neglect of protocol.

Commentary

The resident expressed relief that this was his last rotation of the year and that he would have the opportunity to participate in an in-depth dermatology teaching experience. The only perceived problem was that of dividing his time between patient care in the family practice center and education in the dermatology clinic. However, medical education and practice do not occur in a vacuum. The resident quickly became aware that his ideas about the consultation process were not practiced by the dermatologist. This created a frustration for the resident as to whether or not it was his role to correct the situation.

Until recently, medical schools and residencies have not provided formal courses in medical ethics. It was felt that these matters were taught by example and by being part of the medical process. The only discussions frequently heard were those concerning fee splitting, ghost surgery, euthanasia, and confidentiality. Very little was taught about the doctor–patient and doctor–doctor relationships. In many of these areas, there are not universally accepted ethical or moral principles to be taught, but only the process of inquiry to define what is best for the patient, the community, and the physician.

The consultation process is a frequently used and necessary part of patient care. It is commonly accepted that family physicians utilize consultations and referrals in less than 5 percent of their encounters with patients. In so doing, the primary physician has a role in coordinating patient care with continuity of relationship and information. When properly executed, the consultation process benefits all individuals involved. The patient derives additional aid in the care of his problem. The primary physician gains an ally in the search for accurate diagnosis and treatment as well as a source of reassurance and practical continuing education. The consultant gains an opportunity to practice his science, personal esteem, and financial rewards.

While the expectations from the consultation process are usually met, there are problems that may frequently develop. When the family physician announces to the patient the need for consultation, the patient may fear that he is seriously or hopelessly ill, that the personal physician is no longer interested in taking care of him, or that there will be increased costs for the medical care. The primary physician is frequently concerned as to whether the consultant will support the diagnosis or imply to the patient that poor care has been rendered. There is also a concern that the consultant may not handle the case correctly or promptly return the necessary information along with the patient. Problems for the consultant include not being properly informed by the primary physician of significant history, studies previously performed, or current therapy. An even more frequent dilemma for consultants is ascertaining the degree of responsibility for care of the patient. The consultant may be unsure of whether to initiate procedures without the advice and consent of the primary physician.

In the incident presented, the problem was that a secondary consultation was made without conferring with the primary physician. It is very frustrating for the physician who refers a patient with psoriasis to a dermatologist to discover that the patient is now being seen by a neurologist and an orthopedic surgeon for problems which are unrelated to the original consultation. To be asked by the patient why this was done before hearing about it from the consultant only increases the distress.

One of the functions of the primary physician is coordination of patient care. With input from the patient and the family, the family physician frequently must transfer responsibility to another specialist for the patient's welfare and benefit. This case illustrates an infringement on the generally accepted principle that a consultant should not request a secondary consultation before discussion with the primary physician, who orchestrates total care of the patient. Problems are generated when essential information is not made available to the second consultant about previous investigation and therapy. This can result in duplication of expensive tests and previously unsuccessful therapies. Conversely, the secondary specialist may not know the primary physician, precluding the reciprocal transfer of consultative information concerning the investigation and recommended therapy. If the dermatologist in this incident continues such a practice, the family physician will be offended. Eventually, this practice can interfere with a consultant developing or continuing a strong referral-based practice. The primary physician must feel safe with the consultant or other avenues of referral will be developed.

A second issue arises in the discussion of the best course of action for the resident. While a resident is a free moral agent, it is often inappropriate for the trainee rotating on other services to monitor the ethical practice of his mentor and to take action based upon his own personally developing medical ethic. Such actions might alienate valuable teaching resources. Insight may be gained by discussing such situations with the residency director and other appropriate faculty. If the resident then does not feel that his personal ethic and feelings can coexist with the situation, a responsible course of action should be planned with the residency director.

No record of action is given in this critical incident. If there was resolution, other than to live with the frustration, we are not informed. A possible solution is that the resident could volunteer to phone the referring physician to inquire whether the problem had been previously treated and whether any investigative studies had been accomplished. If the problem recurred, the resident could volunteer the same, but in addition make a statement that he also felt the need to get the referring doctor's permission for the secondary consultation. If this prompts a discussion between the resident and the consultant, the resident might then state his personal feelings as to how he would like his patients managed by consultants, especially regarding the generation of secondary consultations without informing the primary physician.

I feel that any further action should be at the discretion of the residency director. He might develop a conference on consultation and invite the offending physician to attend or participate, send copies of consultation protocols to the preceptors in other specialties who train family practice residents, or discuss the situation directly with the involved consultant. The role of the consultant and the primary physician is an excellent topic for the monthly hospital staff meeting. The expectations and problems of both the primary physician and the consultants can be explored and a statement of general rules can be established. There are complementary roles for the primary physician and the consultant. It is necessary that a collaborative relationship be developed for good patient care and physician satisfaction.

Harry E. Mayhew, M.D.
Professor and Chairman
Department of Family Medicine
Medical College of Ohio at Toledo
Toledo, Ohio

Suggested Readings

Bates, R. C. Successful consultation. *Medical Economics,* December 10, 1979, 173–179.

Cummins, R. O., Smith, R. W., & Inui, T. S. Communication failure in primary care. *Journal of the American Medical Association,* 1980, 243(16), 1650–1652.

Geyman, J., Brown, T., & Rivers, K. Referrals in family practice. *Journal of Family Practice,* 1976, 3(2), 163–167.

Saunders, T. C. Consultation-referral among physicians: Practice and process. *Journal of Family Practice,* 1978, 6(1), 123–128.

17 / "The Compazine Affair"
Interprofessional Conflicts in Special Care Units

Background

I was a second-year resident on an ICU service, functioning as an intern once again. It was a rough service with very ill patients, long intensive hours, and, unfortunately, an attending physician who was not very supportive. This attending frequently relied on the information given by the ICU nurses (whom he knew well) rather than the information given by the "interns" and the supervising resident.

This incident began with the admission of a patient who had just been discharged from another hospital, two weeks after a massive infarction of the anterior myocardium, giving rise to an early ventricular aneurysm. He had been doing well at home until he developed some angina-like chest pain and took a nitroglycerin. He promptly passed out and was brought by life squad to the emergency room, where he began to vomit. His vital signs were stable, but since he had ST segment elevations across the precordium on EKG, he was admitted to rule out extension of the previous myocardial infarction.

The Incident

The incident was precipitated by the supervising resident insisting that I give this elderly gentleman an intravenous bolus of 100 mg of lidocaine. I felt this was too large a bolus for an older person. However, the resident insisted. The large bolus was given and the patient promptly began vomiting and developed paresthesias. We finally stabilized the patient and admitted him to the ICU with an intravenous drip of lidocaine at 2 mg per minute. He was still nauseated, so we were allowing him only clear liquids by mouth. At approximately 2:00 A.M., I received a call from an ICU nurse saying that the patient was nauseated and had just vomited. I ordered that the patient be restricted to nothing by mouth and be watched closely. The nurse asked if I would order Compazine to be given for the nausea and I said no.

Fifteen minutes later I received a frantic call from the same nurse saying that the supervising resident had ordered IM Compazine to be given seven minutes ago and now the patient's blood pressure was 60/0 and he was comatose. After a quick burst of profanity on my part, I said that I would be right down and raced to the ICU. The patient was as the nurse described him. Fortunately, he quickly responded to IV fluids and Trendelenburg positioning. After the patient's vital signs stabilized, I notified the supervising resident, who rushed over to the patient and began giving orders to increase the IV rate. I told him that I thought that the Compazine may have been responsible for the hypotensive episode. He naturally disagreed with me, but I let the matter drop since there was a lot of emotion involved at that time.

The patient recovered uneventfully, but I was furious with both the supervising resident and the nurse who had deliberately circumvented my order. (It turned out that she had been unhappy with my refusal to order Compazine and had sought out the supervising resident and asked if he would order Compazine, not telling him what I had said). The next morning I sought out the head nurse of the ICU. After I told her my side of the story, she began to lash out at me, claiming that I was not interested in my patients and that the nurse in question had to actually ask me to come down and take care of the patient when his blood pressure dropped. In addition, she began to tell me that she was not comfortable with a "noncardiologist" (meaning me) taking care of a cardiac patient in the ICU. At this point, I went from angry to livid. With poorly concealed rage, I informed her that I was very angry with nurses circumventing our (the interns') orders on a regular basis and that if they have doubts about our orders, they should bring them up with us directly or with the attending on rounds. I also told her that the nurse on duty the preceding night was lying outright when she stated that she had to insist that I come down to see my hypotensive patient.

Gradually we both calmed down. It turned out that the nurses felt that they should be more involved in the treatment of patients. I agreed to try to involve the nurses more in the treatment plans for the patients. However, I added the reservation that I didn't feel that the nurses should be managing the care of the patients. The head nurse didn't answer; she pursed her lips and turned away.

Discussion

The issue raised in my mind surrounds what to do when a nurse feels that she should manage the patient's care and deliberately circumvents your orders. To what extent should you involve the nurses in the treatment plan for the patient? Was I as negligent of my patient's care as the head nurse claimed? I felt that I was being very diligent in the care of my patients and that my patients were doing very well in general. How do you deal with the resentment you feel when everybody begins to treat you like an intern again? More specifically, what do you do when your supervising resident (who is also a second-year resident with less ICU experience than yourself) insists on your doing things that you feel are inadvisable? How big a fuss should you raise regarding the Compazine incident and the subsequent behavior of the nurse when it is going to put you in conflict with your supervising resident, the nurse on duty, and the head nurse as well?

Commentary

This incident and the questions raised by the resident do not result from a single interaction alone but are symptomatic of changes going on not only in this young resident's life but in medicine itself. Though the resident's personal frustrations literally leap from the page with a force that must certainly demand rational and specific answers, it is to the larger issues that we must address our concern in a search for solutions and advice. Just as family medicine seeks to develop its own identity to instill new force in old principles, so too is the profession of nursing seeking a new identity and a new role in the health care system. For the most part, the principle of team care has been accepted, but with its acceptance a group of principles were necessary for the proper functioning of such team care approaches, and it is these principles which apply to the problem we are currently addressing. The difference in this particular case is that the so-called team is not a formally organized group but a chance coupling of an on-duty resident, supervising resident, and nurse.

Additionally, we have the problem so common to residents and residency training—the need for identity of the residents themselves. This most crucial search is carried on in an atmosphere of pressure, fatigue, and changing perspectives during a period of time when the true responsibility for patient care finally becomes a reality for the neophyte physician. Would that emergencies did not occur at 2:00 A.M., when forces are low and fatigue plays as much a role in the formulation of a plan as good medical judgment.

The resident contests the nurse's statement that she had actually asked the resident to respond in person to care for the patient with hypotension.

Perhaps the words were never spoken, but certainly the intent of the phone call to the resident at that time was for help in the care of this patient, help which could be rendered only in person and after careful examination and consideration of the patient's actual state. The response by the resident to continue observation was insufficient for the needs of the nurse and, therefore, additional help had to be summoned. It would be unfair to lay the total burden upon the resident, who probably was barely roused from a deep and needed sleep when the decision was requested of him. Perhaps the nurse might have been more explicit. However, certainly the failure of the resident to meet with the needs of the nurse at that time form part of this problem. Physician negligence? Probably not—merely faulty perception of the true import of that early morning call. The resident wishes to know what to do about the nurse who deliberately circumvented the orders. Yet the orders were insufficient to the need of both nurse and patient and were not circumvented but rather replaced by what seemed to be a more definitive and positive action. The resulting effect upon the patient is merely incidental to the underlying problem, although I am sure that the spontaneous "burst of profanity" did little to help mitigate the situation during its resolution phase.

The interplay between residents and nurse can be resolved only when certain specific protocols are set in place. These protocols must give clear recognition and appreciation to the skills and abilities of each member of the team. In addition to establishing a set of principles upon which actions may be predicated, such protocols allow each team member to be identified with his own professional identity and enable an appreciation of one team member for the abilities and skills of the others. In such a situation, insecurity is diminished, anxiety is reduced, and turf battles are kept to a minimum. The physician is permitted to assume the roles and responsibilities that are essential for his actions and his involvement in patient welfare.

Communication among all involved is an absolute must; the understanding of the common goals for patient welfare form a solid basis for such lines of communication. Had this resident been better known or had a previous opportunity for establishing his validity as physician existed, the nurse might well have accepted the initial order "to continue observation." Such communications can be accomplished only when there are frequent meetings of those individuals participating in the patient's care and when an opportunity exists for free exchange of ideas and concerns. Conflicts are diminished and the negativism expressed toward the resident, of being a noncardiologist, can be adequately rebutted.

A sign which hangs on the wall in the office of a residency director friend of mine states, "Just because you are paranoid doesn't mean they are not out to get you." Although there is a strain of paranoia in this critical incident report, it does not negate the fact that family practice residents frequently are placed in the position of proving themselves over and over again. It is not good enough to be good; one must be better than that. It is here that the directors of family practice programs must exercise their greatest diplomacy and put forth their finest efforts. It is the duty of the director to resolve this problem in such a way that the conflict which his resident fears will be initiated with both the supervising resident and the nurse on duty as well as the head nurse, in fact, never occurs. Moreover, he should assure that the incident, which proved the medical astuteness of the family practice resident, is utilized to the utmost to prove the validity of his education as well as of the program.

With sensitivities sharpened by such an experience and the opportunity provided for further explanation of the responsibilities and duties of the family practice resident, this incident may well evolve into a positive force for all concerned, including the residency program.

Allan H. Bruckheim, M.D.
Associate Professor of Family Medicine
State University of New York at Stony Brook
Stony Brook, New York

Suggested Readings

Andrus, L. H., O'Hare-Devereaux, M., Singler, R., & Mitchell, F. M. The health care team. In R. B. Taylor (Ed.), *Family medicine: Principles and practice*. New York: Springer-Verlag, 1978.

Bates, B. Doctor and nurse, changing roles and relations. *New England Journal of Medicine*, 1970, *283*, 129.

Polliack, M. R. Teamwork in family medicine. In J. H. Medalie (Ed.), *Family medicine—principles and applications*. Baltimore: Williams & Wilkins, 1978.

Wise, H. The primary health care team. *Archives of Internal Medicine*, 1972, *130*, 438.

Commentary

Although this critical incident could be labeled The Compazine Affair and the Liar, the incident demonstrates merely the tip of the iceberg of hostilities and conflict which occur between physicians and nurses, physicians and physicians, and physicians, nursing, and/or hospital administration within a bureaucratic and hierarchical institutional atmosphere. The lack of medical, nursing, and hospital administration leadership is evidenced through questions raised by the resident regarding the extent to which ICU nurses should manage patient care and circumvent medical orders; the head nurse's accusations of negligent medical care by the resident; the complete putdown and total stripping of the resident's authority by the supervising resident and the head nurse; and a chief of service who "sides with the head nurse." The final dilemma is one of professional judgment regarding what is right for the patient. The "intern," who is still performing in an educational capacity, is weighing the decision of whether to make a fuss about the Compazine administration or let the matter drop and, thus, not rock the boat.

The resident readily admitted that he was functioning in anger and hostility at having his medical orders overruled by the supervising resident at the time of the patient's admission. Then, following the administration of the Compazine against his (the resident's) order, the supervising resident also supported the order for Compazine. At least the family practice resident recognized his angered state at the time of the 2:00 A.M. incident and reported that he remained "furious with the supervising resident and the nurse who deliberately circumvented his order."

The nurse acted in a most unprofessional manner, was dishonest, and, therefore, a liar. The degree of honesty a person expresses is determined by the amount of security and self-esteem he or she has, which allows him or her to be more or less honest in seeing a situation as it really is. Dishonesty, whether consciously elaborated or unconsciously demonstrated, is a defensive maneuver designed to support a neurotic system. We distinguish between the deliberate and unconscious liar only because we still tend to assign moral judgments to these types of distortions (Salzman, 1976).

Unless some positive action is taken, the hostility this resident feels for the nurses will continue and the quality of patient care may suffer, as this incident has destroyed their future relationship. Truth must be the guiding principle in social intercourse. Lying makes it impossible to derive any benefit from conversation. Liars are, therefore, held in general contempt (Kant, 1976).

In support of the nurses, we do not know the extent of their educational background. (Does this registered nurse have a Masters in Nursing? Is she a prepared clinician?) Nor are we told the length of their graduate practice experiences in nursing, nor the length of time each has been on the nursing staff of this specific unit. We do know that nurses are responsible for care of patients 24 hours a day on each unit and their relationship with the medical staff can control, through the use of "hidden power," the extent and/or rapidity of patient recovery. Major research has demonstrated that one of the most fundamental unresolved issues for nurses is the lack of recognition of their worth in patient care. It is acknowledged that nurses are the primary and cohesive link that binds all of the health professions and the delivery mechanisms in obtaining the ultimate goal—the provision of high-quality care to patients (National Commission on Nursing, 1981).

Unless the conflict created by this incident can be resolved, this resident and future physicians will continue to be educated in a quality-poor environment. To manage the conflict, the resident has suggested one mode of resolution. He is considering confronting the persons involved but realizes there are risks inherent in this approach, especially at this period of his career.

The writer believes that a confrontation process must take place. Confrontation is defined as a systematic process or sequence that is followed by parties who are in conflict and are trying to resolve that conflict (National League for Nursing, 1981).

However, the parties should include not only those involved in "the Compazine incident," but also the chief of service, the director of nursing, the hospital administrator, or their designees. The goal of the conferences should be to seek objective solutions to improve relationships in the ICU and to arrive at consensus decisions that will involve a high level of commitment of both physicians and nurses to high-quality client care.

The resident in the heated exchange with the head nurse, "agreed to involve nurses more in the treatment plans for patients." What could evolve from the suggested broader-based conferences are protocols for collaborative approaches to client care in the unit. Joint or collaborative practice in hospitals refers to jointly determined relationships between physicians and nurses for the purpose of integrating their care into a single comprehensive approach to patients' needs. Joint practice promotes a climate of trust and respect between the two professions based on their explicitly and jointly defined, mutually complementary roles in patient care (The National Joint Practice Commission, 1981).

Initiated through constructive action of this family practice resident could be a standing intensive care unit collaborative practice committee wherein nurses' freedom to exercise individual initiative is limited to a "defined scope of practice" by hospital standards and by state nurse and medical practice acts. Experience shows that fear of "nurses practicing medicine" had no foundation in the project units (The National Joint Practice Commission, 1981).

Including nurses in collaborative decision making in an atmosphere of mutual respect not only fosters a better educational environment and improves quality of care but is, in itself, an evaluation process.

Elsa L. Brown, R.N., Ph.D.
Professor of Nursing
Dean, School of Allied Health
Medical College of Ohio at Toledo
Toledo, Ohio

References

Kant, E. Ethical duties toward others: Truthfulness. In S. Gorovitz, A. Jameton, R. Macklin, J. O'Connor (Eds.), *Moral problems in medicine*. Englewood Cliffs, New Jersey: Prentice-Hall, 1976.

National Commission on Nursing. *Initial report and preliminary recommendations*. Chicago: Author, September 1981.

The National Joint Practice Commission. *Guidelines for establishing joint or collaborative practice in hospitals* (Reprint). Chicago: Neely Printing Co., 1981.

National League for Nursing. *Management of conflict, publication no. 16-1859*. New York: Author, 1981.

Salzman, L. Truth, honesty, and the therapeutic practice. In S. Gorovitz, A. Jameton, R. Macklin, J. O'Connor (Eds.), *Moral problems in medicine*. Englewood Cliffs, New Jersey: Prentice-Hall, 1976.

18 / Who Should Tell the Patient?
A Physician-Nurse Dilemma

Background

It was about 7:00 P.M. on the surgical ward when I got a call from the nurses on another floor informing me that a patient of one of the attending physicians to whom I was assigned had been admitted from the emergency room to my service. I was a first-year family practice resident rotating on the surgical service for the month. My job consisted of taking house call every Thursday plus working up and writing orders on all patients admitted to my attending physician from 7:00 A.M. to 7:00 P.M. and at night when on call. Since it was 7:00 P.M. and since the attending had not been able to evaluate the patient, I hurried to the patient's bed to discover that the patient was a 50-year-old black man who had been seen in the emergency room with bright red blood per rectum. The patient's history was that for about the past eight months he had noticed some spotting in his underpants. He claimed that he had experienced some constipation and diarrhea intermittently during this time and that he had been afraid to see the doctor because he was worried that he might have "something bad." Since it was 7:00 P.M., I hurriedly evaluated the patient, completed the physical examination, and found significantly that the patient had a Blumer's shelf per rectum and bright red rectal bleeding.

Since his hemoglobin and hematocrit seemed stable and it was now 8:00

P.M., I kept him on the general surgical ward. Appropriate orders were written and the problem of rectal bleeding was superficially discussed with the patient, who seemed disinterested, at best, in what was happening to him.

In the chart I wrote that this was "most probably carcinoma" and included the appropriate workup, which included sigmoidoscopy by the attending physician and myself in the morning, followed by barium enema to rule out other causes of rectal bleeding and "to confirm my suspicions of rectal carcinoma." I also felt that it would be better for me to have a definitive diagnosis of cancer before I mentioned this to the patient. I therefore told him that I had felt a mass in his rectum and that this was probably some sort of tumor, but that we should both wait and have it confirmed by the attending physician in the morning. No mention of malignancy or cancer was made to the patient. Since it was nearing 8:30, I went home, signing out to the other surgical resident on call.

The Incident

About midnight on the night of the patient's admission he complained of restlessness and insomnia and asked the nurses for some sleep medication. Since the 15 mg of Dalmane that had been prescribed had been given at 10:00 P.M., the patient's request was denied. According to the nursing staff, the patient then demanded to see his chart. He was told by nurses that it was inappropriate and that they could answer any questions that he might have. At that point a nurse went to the chart, opened it, and read "Impression—rectal bleeding, suspect carcinoma of the rectum," and told that patient that "he most probably had cancer."

The next morning I made rounds with the attending and was confronted by the patient as to why I had not told him about his diagnosis of cancer. The patient was apprehensive, distrustful, agitated, and depressed. The patient was entertaining the idea of suicide in order to avoid the terrible pain that he anticipated as a victim of cancer. It was difficult for the attending and myself to reestablish rapport with this particular patient.

We did a sigmoidoscopy that morning on the reluctant patient and biopsied the lesion. The patient had adenocarcinoma of the rectum. The remainder of the workup was negative for metastases or tumor. The patient was referred to radiotherapy. Surgery and supportive therapy with a psychotherapist were anticipated.

The attending and I realized that the nurse was out of bounds in her reading the chart to the patient and that she could be made liable for actions. But I realized, along with the other residents, who are readily accessible to the nursing staff, that if such an incident was reported, the nursing staff might "retaliate" against us house officers by creating more on-floor problems, such as calling us in the middle of the night to tell us of a slight rise in a patient's temperature, knowing that it was insignificant but that they were able to "pay us back" by waking us up. Therefore, we did not report this nurse in order to avoid "the hassles" of a vengeful nursing staff.

Discussion

The main question I have about this incident is whether I should have reported the nurse. Would the punishment have justified the potential re-taliatory nuisances for the next two years? Other questions are: What should house staff, including myself, tell a patient regarding a suspected diagnosis of cancer when the patient had not been examined by an attending physician? I was, in this instance, although highly suspicious, still doubtful about the diagnosis without sigmoidoscopy and the backup of the attending. What role should the nursing staff have in discussing a diagnosis with a patient? What rights did this patient have, at the time, to demand that his chart be reviewed by a nurse? Should the nurse in question have called the house officer on call? And, if so, what was his obligation to the patient? How could this entire situation have been avoided by better communication?

Commentary

There are a number of ethical dilemmas in this critical incident. The main question put forth was whether the nurse should have been reported. Far more important is how the situation could have been avoided and how similar incidents can be avoided in the future.

It appears the major question revolves around issues of control, ego, and territory: Is the hospitalized patient just the physician's patient? Does the nurse have any independent responsibility for a patient? The fact that the attending and the resident talked about making the nurse liable for their actions suggests that neither of them was primarily interested in patient care but rather in the power struggle.

The resident states that while he discussed the problem of rectal bleeding with the patient, the patient seemed disinterested, at best, with what was happening to him. The patient was told that this was probably some type of tumor and that further investigation would take place in the morning. Nothing was mentioned to the patient about the possibility of cancer. Because the resident was working late, it was probably a welcome relief that the patient did not raise any questions about the word *tumor*.

The anger that the patient displayed the next morning appears to be similar to that described by Kübler-Ross (1969) in her book *On Death and Dying*, but the resident intimates that the patient's anger was directly attributable to the nurse's professional indiscretion. Further on, the resident commented that supportive therapy with a psychotherapist was anticipated; once again the inference is that this was necessary because of the nurse's mistake. Neither of these assumptions can be justified, since the patient might easily have responded in the same manner when he was told he had cancer after the investigation of his problem.

The major point is how this situation could have been prevented and similar situations can be prevented in the future. Communication by way of the chart among the various persons involved in patient care is of vital importance. The Problem-Oriented Medical Record of Lawrence Weed, M.D., has a specific area under the "Plan" for recording patient education (Hurst and Walker, 1972). If the resident had indicated in the problem-oriented note under "Patient Education" what the patient had been told (and in this case what the patient had not been told), the incident could have been avoided.

Whether a house officer should tell a patient of his suspected diagnosis prior to a discussion with the attending physician depends on the resident's knowledge of the attending. If the resident is comfortable handling the problem in the manner of the attending, he or she should properly proceed. If not, the attending should be called and asked for a specific direction.

In this case telling the patient he had a mass that needed further investigation is a realistic way of handling the problem initially. If the patient questioned more pointedly as to whether or not he had cancer, the resident would have to answer as truthfully as he could, for example, by saying that the possibility exists but further tests and studies would have to be made to rule it out.

The role of the nursing staff in discussing a problem with a patient brings into focus the modern nurse and the new role the nurse plays in patient care. There was a time when the nurse was simply a handmaiden of the physician. With an expanded role, the nurse has come to recognize that he or she has a responsibility to the patient independent of the physician. For example, if a physician chooses not to tell a patient that he has cancer, the nurse who is asked the specific question, "Do I have cancer?" is in an untenable ethical position. If physicians expect the modern nurse to be capable of doing things that are taught today, there needs to be some latitude for decision making on the part of that same nurse.

This nurse had several choices. The one she made was by far the poorest. A telephone call to the covering resident to ask for a repeat of the nighttime sedation would have probably prevented this incident. Instead, she was confronted by an angry patient. Once the patient demanded to see the chart, calling the covering resident to come and talk to the patient would have been an acceptable choice. The resident could then have made the decision about whether to call the attending.

Not reporting the nurse was appropriate. The incident is not of the same magnitude as administering the wrong medication, for example. Reporting

the nurse would have been vindictive, would have done nothing to improve
interprofessional communication and trust, and would probably have brought
on nursing staff retaliation against the house staff. Most important, it would
have done nothing to improve patient care. Reporting the nurse would have
gained nothing except personal satisfaction. The resident's motives would
then have to be questioned.

A private discussion of the incident between the nurse and the resident
would be appropriate. Open communication in an adult–adult manner as
described by Harris (1969) is vital in this interaction. It is important that both
the resident and the nurse gain a better understanding of each other's position
and recognize that they both could have handled their part better.

The major implication of the incident for the practice and training of family
physicians is the importance of recording on the chart what has transpired
between the providers of care and the patient. It is vital. All too often charts
are sketchily filled out. Our involvement with the "subjective" and the
"objective" entries of the problem-oriented medical record leaves little time
or space to record something of equal importance: what the patient has been
told.

Medical education has a challenge to increase communication skills during
a residency program. Too little time is spent improving the interaction
between the residents and other professionals. It is vital that all members of
the health care team be able to communicate openly, while recognizing that
each has an important responsibility for the quality of patient care.

D. Henry Ruth, M.D.
Director, Family Practice Residency Program
Medical Center of Beaver County, Inc.
Beaver, Pennsylvania

References
Harris, T. A. *I'm ok—you're ok*. New York: Harper & Row, 1969.
Hurst, J. W., & Walker, H. K. *The problem-oriented system*. Baltimore:
Medcom Press, 1972.
Kübler-Ross, E. *On death and dying*. New York: Macmillan, 1969.

Commentary

The issue of the patient's right to information and the conditions by which he
may obtain such information has broad implications for professional practice
and the interrelationships between patient, physician, nurse, and other
health care professionals. The issue is one which is now defined by law and all
health professionals must know how to handle such incidents. In the specific

incident described, the handling of the situation was inappropriate by both nurse and physician. The situation is also not representative for this issue of access to information and responsibilities of both nurse and physician.

The nurse exercised a lack of judgment in informing the patient of a probable diagnosis of cancer, a situation which is clearly recognized as being extremely threatening to any patient. Furthermore, it was done after 10 o'clock at night, without access to the physician or complete information. In this action, the nurse demonstrated a lack of competence in not recognizing the patient's state of anxiety and providing supportive care which would clarify his concerns, that is, listen to his feelings and focus his attention on the questions he wished to discuss with his physician the following day. Under the circumstances, the nurse could and should have supported the patient's right to information without providing the information. In the event the patient could not be calmed, the physician should have been called. In essence, the nurse increased the patient's anxiety instead of responding therapeutically.

The physician's response to the situation with the nurse was also inappropriate. His assessment of the situation, that is, "the attending and I realized that the nurse was out of bounds in her reading the chart to the patient and that she could be made liable for actions," was made without any recognition of the factors involved in the situation—the patient's right to information and the skills required to handle an anxious and demanding patient. The only response considered was "punishing" the nurse. More important, the physician avoided the problem—presumably out of fear of retaliation, but most likely out of anxiety in not knowing how to confront the issue and discuss it in a constructive manner. Thus, the stage remains set for a repetition of the problem.

How could the situation have been avoided?

The physician made an accurate assessment of the patient's physical problem and prescribed an appropriate plan of diagnosis while he obtained information regarding the patient's psychological state (avoidance of the problem, worry that it might be "something bad," disinterest in explanations). The physician did not explore this with the patient nor attempt to deal with it. He provided the patient with factual information at a level compatible with the diagnostic process he had developed, then left. The patient remained in the care of the nurse. However, the physician did not discuss the patient's condition or his plan of action with her. A brief consultation would have provided the opportunity to develop a coordinated plan of care.

The role of the nurse in discussing a diagnostic with the patient is well established. Nursing has as its focus of practice the patient's ability to care for himself and the goal of increasing that ability in matters of health. The patient is the recipient of the nurses' care on a mutual contract basis. The nurse is thus expected to respond to the patient *in a therapeutic (helpful) way*, despite the fact that many physicians believe that the nurse has no role in discussing a diagnosis with a patient. This means that the nurse must learn to respond to the patient's request for information, to facilitate his gaining the information, to focus the questions of the patient, and even to validate that which the patient already knows—"I have cancer, don't I?"

In order to function in the patient's care *in a therapeutic way,* the nurse is also required to work collaboratively with the patient's physician and to work toward mutual respect and trust in this collaborative role. In this endeavor she would not take the action described in this incident because it was not therapeutic for the patient and it was not compatible with a collaborative role between respected professionals. Neither did the physician's attitude provide a basis for such a role.

The avoidance of interpersonal confrontations and the lack of skill in knowing how to handle such situations has detrimental effect on the emotional lives of all health professionals—both professionally and personally.

Grace H. Chickadonz, R.N., Ph.D.
Dean and Professor of Nursing
Medical College of Ohio at Toledo
Toledo, Ohio

III / The Patient

The relationship between the family physician and his patient is unique in medicine. Family practice is the only medical specialty in which the physician follows patients throughout the life cycle and is the personal physician for the entire family. The family physician treats the patient and family, not just the disease. Consequently, an intimate bond develops between the family physician and his or her patients. This bond is a double-edged sword. When things go well between doctor and patient, the family physician may experience an immensely gratifying relationship that is not often possible in other medical specialties. However, when difficulties develop in the doctor–patient relationship or when treatment is not successful, that same close relationship can produce frustration and anxiety for the doctor, the patient, and the family. Such strains are critical in that they can negatively affect the outcome of patient care, especially if they lead to noncompliance or termination of the relationship.

In this section, "The Patient," we examine critical incidents and issues that pertain directly to interactions between physicians and patients and/or their families. The first three incidents involve terminally ill patients and their families. Two others describe interactions with patients who have been traditionally labeled "problem patients." The remaining incidents describe less common but extremely difficult management problems: a prejudiced pat-

ient, sexual acting-out on a hospital ward, and conflicts between medical science and the religious beliefs of patients.

A common theme running through these incidents is that the physician has to make immediate decisions relevant to patient care in the midst of situations that produce strong emotional reactions. Some of the incidents are remarkable primarily because of the emotional impact they have on the physician. In others the physician's emotions lead to decisions that ultimately result in the termination of the doctor–patient relationship. In such instances, the commentators usually assert that the physician made an impulsive and erroneous decision. However, the reader must ask himself whether he would be able to show any more flexibility of judgment in the heat of the moment generated by the same situations.

Another theme that runs through many of the incidents is the interactive nature of the doctor–patient relationship. Here, as in the previous section, the question of blame is not relevant to these incidents. Rather, the behaviors, attitudes, and beliefs of both the doctor and the patient contribute to making these situations problematic. Often, it is a conflict between the expectations and needs of the physician and those of the patient and family which gives rise to the difficulties described. In considering these incidents, the reader should ponder what each party might have done differently to prevent these situations from becoming critical incidents.

The Editors

19 / Watch Me Die
A Patient's Refusal of Medical Care

Background

A 60-year-old white male had had an uneventful posterior-wall myocardial infarction six weeks previously. He recently had used his arms to fly a U-controlled model airplane during a very hot and humid morning in August. His wife called at the lunch hour and stated that her husband (our patient described) had suddenly clutched his chest and fallen to the floor and was sweating profusely. I arrived minutes later (the ambulance squad was not called because the husband requested his wife *not* to do so) to find him having, presumably, a second myocardial infarction, with bradycardia and severe pain. After administering atropine and Demerol, within moments I was confronted with the following.

The Incident

My patient and his wife had agreed not to allow admission to the area hospital or to allow any further treatment by me or anyone, medically. They had discussed this together prior to this second attack and she informed me that it would be useless to try to persuade them otherwise. The husband slipped into cardiogenic shock and died peacefully over the next one-and-one-half hours as I sat by his bedside listening, monitoring, and documenting his condition. Death was known as his apparent outcome and no assistance was desired except for pain relief. I respected their wishes and documented all of this.

Discussion

I reported this incident to several other physicians on my hospital staff in both its legal and moral implications. Do we have the right, medically, to restrict care when a possibly salvageable illness occurs, just because the patient and legal survivor request this "no action"?

Commentary

It has been argued consistently and effectively in recent years by moral philosophers and theologicans that patients and their families, acting freely, competently, and informedly, can refuse extraordinary medical interventions merely to prolong life in the face of uncurable and/or terminal medical conditions. As a matter of fact, patients can make this decision in advance and carry on their persons a card conveying this decision to any hospital or doctor. Of course, there is sometimes disagreement as to what interventions qualify as extraordinary, but the principle is established.

The case presented here hardly seems to come under the provisions described. The patient is not aged, debilitated, suffering chronic pain, nor otherwise compromised except by an acute cardiovascular event that, on the surface, seems eminently amenable to treatment with good chance of recovery. The behavior of this couple is so unusual as to be eccentric and raises questions of a suicide pact, severe depression, *folie à deux*, or other abnormal mental states. No rationale is presented that justifies the nontreatment of the patient except the wish for death. An analogous scenario can be imagined if the patient had accidentally severed a major artery while working in his shop and then refused treatment while exsanguinating at home. Surely no physician would accede to a request that the bleeding not be stopped by any means possible.

It is the presence of the doctor that makes this incident morally interesting. If the doctor had not been there, the patient would have become by law a coroner's case and the cause of death, including the possibility of foul play, would have been investigated. Provided the doctor is willing to sign the death certificate, no coroner's inquest is likely to occur and the unusual circumstances of the patient's death will not appear in any official public record. Does the doctor's passive participation in this terminal event make him an accessory in an unlawful death? Worse, does his administration of pain-relieving drug(s) make him a collaborator in the patient's death?

If the patient and his wife had been strangers to the doctor, there seems to be no question but that the doctor would have been obligated to mobilize the emergency care system by calling an ambulance or the police or both, because there would have been no basis for the couple's appeal to do nothing. They were not strangers, however, since the doctor was presumably involved in the treatment of the first infarct six weeks before, and it is that relationship that allows the couple to prevail. This seems to me to be an abuse of the relationship on the part of the couple and an inappropriate surrender on the part of the doctor. In the absence of mitigating circumstances, which we are not given, the doctor should have taken unilateral action to get the patient to a hospital, even over the protests of the couple. This might have meant calling the police.

This is the safest course for the doctor since I can imagine no legal recriminations from such action. On the other hand, the doctor could be vulnerable to later litigation by a grief-stricken wife or some other family member based on the allegation that the doctor did not act prudently to save life. The very strangeness of this incident would alert me to the possibility that stranger things could occur and that suing me might be one of them. I would hate to be in a court with the wife as an accusor and be without other witnesses, having as my only defense that the couple insisted on "no action." I would rather trust that no court would convict me for trying to save the man.

The larger issue raised by this incident concerns the right to die in our society. On the whole the law is careful to uphold the sanctity of life and guards the circumstances in which death is permissible. All medically unattended deaths are investigated by the authorities, and medically attended deaths require documentation by a physician, who, in such instances, acts as a civil authority. The taking of life by any means is unlawful except after due process, and contributing to the death of another is also unlawful. Suicide and euthanasia are no exceptions. Physicians are constrained by both the law and medical tradition to save life, and exceptions to this are carefully guarded.

Persons unattended by physicians can do a great deal to hasten their deaths by refusing to eat, ingesting drugs and alcohol, and failing to seek medical care all without legal recriminations—unless they happen to be the subject of complaints by family, friends, or neighbors. Once there is a medical attendant, however, the responsibility for life is shifted toward the professional and the patient is no longer free to decide his fate in isolation. Physicians should not be intimidated by patients or compelled by sympathy to contribute to their patients' deaths.

G. Gayle Stephens, M.D.
Professor and Chairman
Department of Family Practice
University of Alabama in Birmingham School of Medicine
Birmingham, Alabama

Commentary

As noted by the physician, this case raises both ethical and legal questions. The focus of this discussion will be primarily on the ethical questions, although the legal issues will be dealt with briefly.

There are two major ethical questions raised by this case. First, what are the limits, if any, of patient autonomy in the situation cited? And second, does respecting the patient's wishes not to receive medical treatment constitute a callous disregard for the value of life by the physician?

The physician was questioning whether he or she had acted appropriately by following the wishes of the patient and his wife in not calling the ambulance to take the patient to the hospital to try to save his life following his second myocardial infarction. The physician seemed uneasy in his or her decision since the patient's situation was viewed as possibly "salvageable." By following the patient's wishes, the physician chose to respect the patient's autonomy, that is, the patient's right to determine what treatment would or would not be accepted.

The information provided in the incident leaves many important questions unanswered; notably, how well did the physician know the patient and what were the patient's reasons for refusing treatment? However, what is described is a considered decision, not an impulsive spur-of-the-moment decision made under the stress and pain of a myocardial infarction. The situation certainly can be described as a medical emergency; but it had been anticipated by the patient and his wife.

There seems to be no question about the mental competence of the patient, which means he had every right to choose the extent of treatment he would or would not accept.

Paternalistic interventions, that is, attempts by the physician to override the patient's instructions, could lead to charges of battery being filed against the physician. This does not mean that the physician should not try to determine why the patient has chosen not to allow hospital treatment in a situation in which his life might be saved, although there are no guarantees that he would live. The physician has an obligation to try to learn how and why this decision was reached. From a legal perspective, it seems that the physician was on solid ground in his or her decision, provided he or she had informed the patient and his wife that the expected outcome in the given situation was death. To go against the patient's decision, which had been made before this incident occurred and which had been discussed with his wife, would appear to have greater potential for legal ramifications than respecting the patient's wishes. Little information is given regarding the physician–patient relationship in the case, but this relationship is often an important determinant in whether or not legal charges are filed against a physician. The physician in this case acted in a caring, thoughtful manner by staying with the patient and administering medications to relieve pain during the last hours of life. The physician carefully documented all that was done for the patient.*

This commentator believes that respect for people demands respect for decisions made by competent adults, especially those decisions specifying the extent of medical treatment to be accepted. (Emergencies are a different class of situations—at least emergencies where prior decisions have not been made. For example, a person in an auto accident who is brought to the emergency room in extreme pain and demanding to die may be treated since the circumstances—extensive blood loss, shock, and pain—warrant emergency interventions. If at a later time, after the situation has become stable, the patient explains reasons for refusing treatment and if the patient is a competent adult, those wishes must be heard and respected.) An argument frequently used to counter the notion that a patient should be allowed to refuse treatment is that such action devalues life and engages the physician in an action contrary to his or her professional purpose, which is to save life. In fact, a counterargument could be that the physician was showing great respect for the patient and not displaying a callous disregard for life.

Obviously the situation in which a patient declines potentially lifesaving treatment will be emotionally difficult for the physician and others involved in the patient's care. There will be situations in which the physician may feel certain that the wrong decision is being made, yet even at these times the patient's right to self-determination demands respect. Deference to the patient's wishes reflects a sensitivity toward the patient as a person and ought not be viewed as a diminution of the value of life.

Joy D. Skeel, B.S. Nsg., M. Div.
Instructor in Medical Humanities, Department of Psychiatry
Instructor in Medicine, Department of Medicine
Medical College of Ohio at Toledo
Toledo, Ohio

---

*It is impossible to document the precise legal ramifications for the physician in this case without knowing the state in which it occurred and the individual state laws pertaining to the situation. My attempt, however, is to articulate the relevant considerations which any physician or court should consider in a case such as the one cited.

20 / "Does God Need Thanks?"
A Grieving Family Rejects the Physician

Background

Early in 1974 my patient, a 29-year-old mother of three, the youngest of whom I had delivered three years previously, presented complaining of fresh rectal bleeding. Investigation included a barium meal, which was reported as "equivocal even with double contrast examination, please repeat in six weeks." I conveyed this to my patient who agreed to the repeat procedure.

She did not come and I did not remember to call her.

In April 1975 she presented again, complaining of abdominal pain, and examination revealed multiple palpable abdominal masses. A laparotomy demonstrated inoperable metastatic cancer of the descending colon, and she was discharged from the hospital a week later, to die.

The Incident

The first day home I visited her; she looked desperately ill, yellow, dehydrated, cachetic. She complained of severe abdominal pain. I decided to inject her with morphine in the expectation that she would die that day.

I was surprised, on my return that evening, to find her sitting up in bed eating bread and butter, looking much better. This seemed an opportune moment to talk with the family and the patient, so I assembled them in the bedroom and opened up the issue by asking them what they understood about the mother's illness.

To my surprise, I was frustrated. There was an immediate unspoken agreement in the whole family that this issue would not be dealt with, at least by me! I left the consultation feeling somewhat inadequate, but accepting the right of these people to deny or accept the situation.

Next day, Mrs. B. had deteriorated again, and the morphine injection was repeated with the same result.

This woman survived seven months, during which time I visited her every evening between 9 and 11 P.M. to give morphine. A district nurse gave the morphine in the mornings. When I visited the home I was always aware of a strangeness, a kind of false acceptance of and heartiness toward me. The husband watched me closely, in a suspicious manner, as I drew up the morphine. I assumed that he was anxious that I might slip in an overdose.

Repeated hints that we could talk were always rebuffed.

In early January I left on vacation, and while I was away I heard that Mrs. B. had died.

The day I returned to work I visited the home, in the evening, casually, and to my shock, the widower was not pleased to see me, admitted me ungraciously and gave strong "go-away" messages.

I felt hurt and rejected, for hadn't I given a part of every evening for seven months to this family? How come they didn't recognize my altruism? (I should add that there were no fees for these visits since they were working-class people without insurance coverage.)

Next came sadness. I felt a real loss of this woman with whom, despite this prolonged relationship, I had never gotten close—I thought, due to her husband's interference.

The last stage for me was anger, when I learned three weeks later that the husband had not only changed to my partner for medical care, but also had overcharged my wife for a small task he had done by chance arrangement in my home.

I felt outraged by his rejection, invaded by his overcharging, and decided that never again was I going to allow this level of dependence (probably both ways).

Discussion

Why should this man be so hostile to me? Reflecting, I suspect he felt at some level a cuckold. Here was this apparently untroubled, competent, educated young doctor doing things for and to his wife which he could not do. And I seemed, with my morphine, to be keeping her alive (a phenomenon I have noted on other occasions). And we know dependency breeds rage.

Did I kill this woman by going on vacation? Did the husband see me as a murderer? Does God need thanks? This one did and still burns because he didn't get them.

After 17 years in practice I think I can easily forgive patients for not getting better, but I still have difficulty when they won't recognize and acknowledge my altruism.

Commentary

The physician in this incident would do well to be aware of the very complex systems that are inherent in grief reactions. Several authors have written about the stages of grief (Lindemann, 1944; Schoenberg, Carr, Kutscher, Peretz, & Goldberg, 1974). Although they may differ somewhat in the numbers and the names of the various stages of grief, present to some degree in all grief reactions are denial, anger, and guilt. One can assume that the husband of a 29-year-old woman who dies of a cancer that was originally not diagnosed by a physician will manifest strongly the feelings of anger, no matter how altruistic the physician may be in attentiveness or in the provision of free services. His hostility might realistically be expected rather than come as a surprise. It may also be well for the physician to note that the response to grief experienced by the husband and by himself may be out of synchrony at a specific point in time. For example, the husband may be engaged in denial when the physician is attempting readjustment, or the husband may be angry when the physician is depressed. The death of a loved one is an example of extreme stress wherein interpersonal relationships tend to become more complex than in normal nonstressful interchange. In this case, we have multiple stresses bearing on the relationship between the husband and the physician.

The grief reaction of the physician—an emotional response outside his conscious control—is also of great importance in this instance. His question "Why should this man be so hostile to me?" indicates that he has not been able to divorce himself from the emotional trauma that the relationship incurred. His question "Did I kill this woman by going on vacation?" is evidence of a feeling of guilt at a time when the husband was in the stage of hostility (anger). Logic would have it that the vacation had nothing to do with the death, but that she died of her malignancy. The real feeling of guilt might be due to the lack of a definitive diagnosis when cure might still have been possible. Although from the radiologist's view the advice was adequate, the family physician should have accepted it as only "advice" and decided whether other diagnostic procedures would have been indicated rather than waiting for further x-rays. This is particularly true since the possible consequences of delay in a case like this are so devastating.

The lack of sigmoidoscopy or colonoscopy in this case represents less than optimal care, given the symptoms and the equivocal radiology report. Although the radiologist recommended repeat x-rays in six weeks, the physician should have arrived at an earlier diagnosis, if at all possible, considering the dire consequences of a delay. One may assume that the patient might deny the possibility of serious illness and neglect to have the studies repeated in six weeks if it were left to her initiative. With this consideration, some sort of fail-safe mechanism needs to be in effect to prevent patients from neglecting follow-up studies.

Whether the physician should provide hundreds of dollars of free service to a patient because "they were working-class people without insurance coverage" is a separate issue. My own feeling is that a *reduced* cost might be justified, but a physician is undervaluing his abilities if he does not charge for his professional services. While the overall cost of the illness to this unfortunate family must have been very high, a reduced fee to cover costs seems reasonable. Free services over a prolonged period of time places a moral burden on the patient and her family which cannot be repaid. This burden can explain why the family did not recognize the physician's altruism.

There are several implications in this case for the practice of family medicine. The family physician must be a total health care deliverer, using laboratory and x-ray studies as they apply to a specific case. He or she may obtain help from practitioners of other specialties as well as help from community health sources, nurses, the legal profession, and the various religious bodies. The family physician, however, must accept the responsibility of comprehensive health care for those patients who come to him. In a situation of such potential danger as this, further diagnostic tests would have been indicated at the time that the first symptoms appeared. I am aware of the concept that the patient is basically responsible for his or her own health care and that, in this incident, a case might be made for the woman herself being responsible for her demise since she did not follow the physician's advice to have her x-rays repeated in the next six weeks. One would have to have more information relative to the understanding between the doctor and the patient at the time of the discussion of the x-rays in order to pursue this point further. The concept of informed consent enters here since one would assume that the physician had explained to her the risks of waiting even six weeks for further tests in contrast to having them at that time or not at all. If she were to be the decision maker, there should be evidence that she was fully informed of the benefits and risks of her decision.

This incident also raises the issue of the role of the patient's religion in medical care. The only reference to God was the question "Does God need thanks?" The physician was referring to *himself* as God if I read the question correctly. What about the religion of the patient and her family? Could not their beliefs have been used constructively? Shouldn't the physician be instrumental in addressing the religious beliefs of the family? Perhaps he did, but the incident as reported does not indicate that this aspect of the care of the patient was addressed at all. Whether the physician was a religious person or not is not the issue. Supporting the religious beliefs of the family is an integral part of the comprehensiveness of care espoused by family physicians.

It is clear that an understanding of the psychodynamics of the relationship between the stages of grief on the part of both the physician and the husband would help answer some of the questions posed in this incident. Training in residency programs in family medicine has progressed to include the behavioral sciences, not formerly part of medical training. Special courses in the behavioral sciences which include seminars, workshops, role-playing, audiovisual feedback, and specific patient care situations are an integral part of family practice residency programs. In these courses the issues addressed in this incident are discussed. This is where the doctor in training learns about the stages of grief, about interpersonal relationships, about accepting him- or herself as a trained physician but certainly not as God. In this one area lies the major difference between the family physician and the general practitioner or other specialist. It is worthy of note that other primary care residencies are beginning to include the behavioral sciences in their training programs. It seems to be a basic requirement for the complete physician (AMA Committee on Graduate Medical Education, 1980).

The review of this case has helped me as a teacher of family practice residents to understand better what we are about in residency programs. Not only competence in diagnosis and therapy are required for the excellent physician, but an understanding of the psychosocial responses to death on the part of both relatives and the doctor must be a part of successful training for the family physician. The behavioral sciences offer a critically important addition to the basic medical training of young family physicians.

Lynn A. Phelps, M.D.
Associate Professor, Family Medicine and Practice
University of Wisconsin
Madison, Wisconsin

References

American Medical Association Committee on Graduate Medical Education. *1980–1981 Directory of residency training programs*. Chicago: AMA, 1980.

Lindemann, E. Symptomatology and management of acute grief. *American Journal of Psychiatry*, 1944, *101*, 141.

Schoenberg, B., Carr, A., Kutscher, A., Peretz, D., & Goldberg, I. *Anticipatory grief*. New York & London: Columbia University Press, 1974.

Commentary

A physician who has been in practice for 17 years asks the question, "Did I kill this woman by going on vacation?" I sense this physician is not asking a question at all, but stating a feeling which troubles him after he cared for this young woman with terminal cancer when he was perceived by her as an "apparently untroubled, competent, educated young doctor." The question of whether the husband saw the physician as guilty of murder or some other sin will be discussed later and relates to the first question. The last question asking "Does God need thanks? This one did" raises the issue of this physician's concept of his role and responsibilities as a physician.

I believe the basis of the many issues raised by this incident is the physician–patient relationship which developed. I can understand the normal mixture of strong feelings in a physician facing the task of managing the care of a 30-year-old mother of three with inoperable metastatic cancer of the descending colon. However, I believe this incident indicates this physician's lack of understanding of his role in the doctor–patient relationship. This is exemplified by his isolating the care of the patient by making daily house calls for several months, feeling guilty about charging for these services, believing this care was curative, developing a relationship with the woman which he perceived as threatening to her husband, and finally feeling outrage at the patient and her husband for not recognizing and acknowledging his altruism. The final implication was that this physician, as God, did need thanks and was not receiving thanks.

For a physician, the fear of failure can lead one to alter, abandon, usurp, misrepresent, or mystify the role of physician. These methods often relieve the anxiety and fear of the physician at the expense of the patient and his or her family. This type of defense in a vulnerable situation soon becomes a habit for allowing the physician to continue in practice and maintain a "sane" position in life.

The responsibilities of the family physician have been covered well by Hiram B. Curry, M.D., in Chapter 4 of *Family Medicine* by Taylor. Regarding the challenges facing the family physician, Dr. Curry states:

> I now believe the major responsibilities of the physician are similar to those of other professionals and other persons in every aspect of life. The nature of the work we do, the role we cast ourselves in, the role we encourage our patients and society to see us in, create a facade that is at once a joy and a curse. It is a joy because we hold a prestigious position and we are accorded respect automatically. Many privileges come to us because we are physicians. It is a curse because there is danger in really believing that we do often hold the lives of our patients in the palms of our hands. It may have been necessary to see one's self cast in this omnipotent role in order to work the long and irregular hours which some physicians endured in the past [Taylor, 1978].

In *The Fortunate Man—The Story of a Country Doctor*, the question is raised:

> How is it that Sassall [the physician] is acknowledged as a good doctor? By his cures? This would seem to be the answer. But I doubt it. You have to be a startlingly bad doctor and make many mistakes before the results tell against you. In the eyes of the layman the results always tend to favour the doctor. No, he is acknowledged as a good doctor because he meets the deep but unformulated expectation of the sick for a sense of fraternity. He recognizes them. Sometimes he fails—often because he has missed a critical opportunity and the patient's suppressed resentment becomes too hard to break through—but there is about him the constant will of a man trying to recognize.
>
> This can be by the doctor presenting himself to the patient as a comparable man. It demands from the doctor a true imaginative effort and precise self-knowledge. . . . It is the doctor's acceptance of what the patient tells him and the accuracy of his appreciation as he suggests how different parts of his life may fit together, it is this which then persuades the patient that he and the doctor and other men are comparable because whatever he says of himself or his fears or his fantasies seems to be at least as familiar to the doctor as to him. He is no longer an exception. He can be recognized and this is the prerequisite for cure or adaptation.
>
> Now the patient is the central character. He tries to recognize each patient and, having recognized him, he tries to set an example for him—not a morally improving example, but an example wherein the patient can recognize himself [Berger & Mohr, 1967].

It is strange that we physicians tend to make the physician–patient relationship very mystical and thereby not involve the patient. The challenge of family physicians is to educate patients of their role in health care so that they may recognize themselves during periods of "dis-ease."

Richard M. Baker and Donald M. Cassatta have provided the elements and concepts of the physician–patient relationship in Chapter 18 in *Family Medicine*. They state:

> Cooperation between the patient and physician usually requires an attitude on both parts that the patient is responsible for his own health management. The physician who usurps this basic responsibility will likely be frustrated and less effective. The patient who attempts to abrogate this basic responsibility will likely be poorly satisfied and less successful in managing his health problems [Taylor, 1978].

The physician in this critical incident was unable to look at his own reality and feelings and attain sufficient self-knowledge to help the patient and her husband recognize themselves in this tragic situation. The physician was unable to turn to others in consultation as a resource. This might have offered the opportunity to begin to look at the dependency relationship which developed. The possibility is alluded to that the physician was receiving secondary gain in the approach he used. Therefore, he would not reflect on the complex interactions and transactions that were occuring until the final rejection by the widower when the physician "casually visited the home." At that point, the feelings became evident and the physician was placed in the role of victim by the persecuting husband. This was uncomfortable compared to the usual rescuer role that the physician had assumed.

This commentary has attempted to understand the comparable situation of this physician and thereby has included many assumptions that may or may not have been someone's perception of the reality of the time.

A person entering the practice of medicine often perceives it as a "calling" and assumes a parent or "God-like" role. The skills required to recognize this tendency, educate the patient to accept the responsibility for his or her own health, and manage the planning for the patient's ongoing health care continue to challenge those of us involved in family medicine.

Charles E. Morrill, M.D.
Director, Grand Rapids Family Practice Residency
Saint Mary's Hospital
Grand Rapids, Michigan

References

Berger, J., & Mohr, J. *A fortunate man—the story of a country doctor*. London: Writers and Readers Publishing Cooperative, 1967.
Taylor, R. B. *Family medicine—principles and practice*. New York: Springer-Verlag, 1978.

Suggested Readings

Froelick, R. E., & Bishop, F. M. *Clinical interviewing skills* (3rd ed.). Saint Louis: Mosby, 1977.
Stephens, G. G. Family medicine as a counter culture. *Family Medicine Teacher*, Summer 1979, 6(5), 14–19.

21 / "Didn't You Examine His Heart?"

Myocardial Infarction following a Normal Evaluation

Background

I have known Mrs. F. for two years. When she first came in to see me as a patient, I identified four problems which needed major consultation: (1) bilateral cataracts, referred to an ophthalmologist; (2) severe vaginal stenosis with no history of surgery or radiation, referred to a gynecologist; (3) weakness of the right leg with some atrophy, diagnosed as peripheral neuritis, etiology unknown, referred to a neurologist; and (4) absence of pulses in the left leg, referred to a peripheral vascular surgeon.

Since that time, I have met her husband, brother, and daughter-in-law. With each individual I have again encountered major illnesses, including sepsis and shock, leg amputation, active duodenal ulcer, alcoholism, breast abcess, and carcinoma of the larynx.

The Incident

Three days ago I saw Mrs. F.'s husband for a general checkup concerning his post-radiation of the cancer of the larynx and healing of his tracheostomy, emphysema, and duodenal ulcer. At no time did the patient discuss difficulty with chest pain. His main complaint was weakness and hoarseness. Examination was negative except for the healing ostomy in his trachea and a few scattered ronchi and increased expiratory breathing in his lungs.

Today I received a call from Mrs. F., who was distraught. Last evening, her husband got up from eating, clutched his chest, and fell over. The rescue squad was called. He was unconscious when he left the home. He was in the coronary intensive care unit at a hospital other than the two in which I practice. After she informed me of this tragic occurrence, she then asked, "Didn't you examine his heart?" I then had several thoughts and feelings that seemed to run through me simultaneously. I felt that I was being blamed for something beyond my responsibility or control. I felt that she was blaming me for his disease. I felt that she implied that I had not practiced good medicine. I felt guilty that I was not able to immediately stop my present duties and rush 14 miles to visit him in the intensive care unit. I felt that she was ignorant of what physicians can know and predict.

At first I listened to her. There were times when I felt I wanted to justify myself and make such statements as "electrocardiograms cannot predict the future," "just because a patient is well today does not assure that he will be the same tomorrow," and "the manifestations of coronary artery disease are often sudden and fatal, giving no warning."

All I was able to state was that I was sorry that it happened and please keep me informed by phone. On reflection, this seemed inadequate and empty.

Discussion
Many times in medicine there are errors of commission and omission which result in guilt. But equally difficult are the feelings which sometimes arise even when the situation was handled correctly and the only problem was being there.

How can I react appropriately when I am shocked, upset, or angry? How can I learn to accept the limits of my responsibility?

Commentary

Upon reading this critical incident, this commentator has an immediate feeling of sympathy and understanding of the physician's reactions, but let us go beyond these feelings and try to analyze the incident to see what can be learned from it.

In analyzing the situation, let us consider it first from Mrs. F.'s point of view, then from the physician's. I shall start with the patient's wife, the complainant or the "accusor," as she is made out to be in this incident. This is, I believe, a vital first step, because unless we empathize with and understand our patients, it is extremely difficult to handle our own reactions as physicians.

From the Patient's Point of View
Mrs. F. is a woman with multiple serious problems and diseases which have already necessitated her being referred to four different subspecialists within two years. The problems with her eyes and legs probably limit her vision and

mobility to a considerable extent. The members of her family that the physician has seen (unfortunately no information is given concerning the family tree, the members of the household, and the human and material resources the family has at its disposal) are people with serious chronic illnesses. This includes her husband, who has one major life-threatening advanced disease (cancer of the larynx which necessitated a tracheostomy) as well as emphysema and a duodenal ulcer. For Mrs. F., with her chronic disabling conditions, to be a support and perhaps even the main caretaker of her husband and to be constantly aware of his tracheostomy, his breathing, his voice, and his weakness must have placed a considerable burden on her already weakened condition. Judging too by the other members of the family known to the physician (one with an amputated leg, another a chronic alcoholic), there is very little likelihood of Mrs. F. receiving too much support from relatives. This leaves her physician as perhaps the one stable and trustworthy support system in her severely stressed and precariously balanced life situation. Then suddenly, her husband, a few days after a general checkup from which he emerged presumably feeling that everything was all right (it would be helpful to know exactly what the physician had told him and his wife and also what examinations were performed), collapses and goes into a coma, presumably as a result of a myocardial infarction or severe arrhythmia.*

Mrs. F.'s initial reaction must have been one of shock and disbelief. After her husband was in the coronary care unit she probably went through some of the subsequent stages of acute separation anxiety tinged with feelings of guilt. Had she done something to contribute to his attack? Very soon another dynamic process comes into play—feelings of hostility, perhaps against her husband, but as is often the case, directed against the physician. This hostility is based on both rational and irrational ideas and thoughts, in this case a mixture of: Did the physician do an EKG? ("Didn't you examine his heart?") plus the perception or misconception of the meaning of the assurance the physician gave Mr. F. after the checkup. In this situation too, Mrs. F.'s feelings are probably very ambivalent: anger at what she thinks the doctor did wrong as well as perhaps fear of antagonizing and losing her main "support system." In the situation described, Mrs. F.'s feelings and actions are understandable and must be allowed for.

---

*The patient's symptoms could have been caused by a sudden perforation of the cancerous process into another organ or space such as the pleural cavity, esophagus, etc. For the purpose of this discussion, we will presume that having been admitted to a coronary intensive care unit, he had suffered a myocardial infarction. In essence, the exact diagnosis does not materially affect the reactions of the two main participants at the time the incident occurred.

From the Physician's Point of View

It is only natural that if the physician is young and inexperienced or has not been through a similar situation during his residency, he will probably not understand or identify with the woman's reactions and therefore will himself go through a series of very similar reactions, including:

1. Shock at the news and, for a few fleeting seconds, perhaps even denial.
2. Anxiety and guilt: Did he miss something in the examination; perhaps he did not do something he should have done; or even if the examination was complete, did he lead them to understand that everything was all right, instead of explaining that within the limitations of the examination nothing abnormal was detected?
3. Anger and hostility: Part of this is turned toward himself and his discipline, but soon it is turned against the woman. Why doesn't she understand? Why is she so unreasonable? After all he has done for her and her family in the last few years—what ingratitude! These feelings will turn inward resulting in a feeling of self-pity. He begins to feel sorry for himself and might even become a little depressed if this phase lasts too long.
4. Attempts at adjustment: This might take the form of asking his colleagues for support, followed by advice as to methods of coping with similar situations in the future.

I believe the physician in question went through some or all of the above phases.

Having explained and understood the reactions of the woman and the physician, I will now try and answer the physician's questions of how to react in a similar situation or, perhaps better, the situation under discussion, knowing, however, that it is easier to be a Monday morning quarterback than the actual player.

When Mrs. F. called, it would take some moments for the physician to recover from the shock of the unexpected news and the physician (as he or she did) would listen while Mrs. F. gave vent to her feelings.

At that stage I believe there are three things to do:

1. Show Mrs. F. that you understand and even identify with her feelings.
2. Defer the discussion of her husband's checkup to a more appropriate time.
3. Show her that your primary concern is your patient in the CCU and make appropriate plans to monitor his condition.

The conversation might have gone something like this:

"Mrs. F., your news is very upsetting and I fully understand your concern about your husband as well as your anger with me. I would probably feel the same in your place. About your husband's checkup examination, this is not the time to discuss it because my immediate concern is your husband. I shall immediately contact the physician in charge of the CCU at X Hospital and will call you back as soon as possible."

Note: In the description of the event, the physician, I believe, retreated from his responsibility for his patient by asking Mrs. F. to keep him informed of his progress. With the anger that Mrs. F. has, I doubt that she would feel inclined to do this.

At that stage, the physician should (whatever the pressures of his workload) speak to the CCU and then call Mrs. F. If, however, the patient had in the meantime died, I think a home visit to Mrs. F. with a face-to-face encounter would be a necessity. The doctor should also make arrangements to visit the CCU either that day, that evening, or the following morning so as to monitor his patient's progress and consult with the treating physician even though he would not be involved in the day-to-day management. At a later date the questions arising out of the checkup examination could be discussed.

The training that family practice residents undergo should help them understand the reactions of patients and physicians to sudden unexpected events. With this understanding, we should hopefully be able to go from the shock stage directly into the adjustment phase. An important part of the latter must be action concerning the patient and his or her family. We should not waste time or energy on our feelings of guilt or anger at the initial contact with the patient or family, although these feelings will probably come to the surface that night or some other time when the physician has time to reflect on his practice. Having done something about the situation, however, the feelings of guilt, and the like, will be minimal. One can sympathize with the physician in the incident, but taking the "long view," it will be a good thing for his or her own development toward becoming a well-rounded family physician if he or she learns from this how to cope better with "unexpected crises" in the future. We have all had to go through similar experiences.

Jack H. Medalie, M.D., M.P.H.
Dorothy Jones Weatherhead Professor and Chairman, Family Medicine
School of Medicine
Case Western Reserve University
Cleveland, Ohio

22 / "I Don't Want Any Nigger Taking Care of Me"
The Prejudiced Patient

Background
I had a private patient on the teaching service with chronic intrinsic asthma.
He was a very hostile, angry, and difficult patient who wheezed when frustrated, depressed, or anxious. At times, his asthma was life-threatening and
required IV steroids, aminophylline, and a respirator. Whenever his wheezing became severe, he would become demanding and panicky, often acting
inappropriately because of frequent near-fatal episodes of asthma. The first-year resident on the service was a black man who came from a small town in
Georgia. He felt out of place in the urban center and was very sensitive about
his color and rural background. He was one of two black residents out of 24
family practice residents in a hospital with very few black employees and even
fewer black patients.

The Incident
At 2 A.M., the patient was admitted via the emergency room with acute
asthma. He was in his usual state of panic with severe air hunger and marked
cyanosis. The resident immediately went to his room with an IV setup for
administration of steroids and aminophylline. When he informed the patient
that he was a doctor and was going to treat his acute asthma, the patient told
him to get out of his room. When the resident persisted in trying to help him,

he shouted, "Get out of here, boy. I don't want any nigger working on me." To which the resident replied, "Suit yourself, man. You can goddam die for all I give a shit." The head nurse then called me and asked what should be done. I came to the floor within two minutes only to be greeted by a furious resident, who stated, "You can take that son-of-a-bitch and treat him yourself, honkey, I'm leaving. I don't have to take this white man bullshit."

I started the IV, administered the epinephrine, Decadron, and aminophylline and sat with the patient until he was comfortable. As I was leaving, his parting comment was, "Thanks a lot, doc, I almost died. But I don't want any nigger taking care of me."

Discussion

How does one deal with prejudice in medicine, whether it be against blacks, foreign graduates, or female physicians? Do you treat the patient, the maligned, or yourself? Who gets priority?

How can you defuse an acute inflammatory situation between a patient and a physician which is based on pure prejudice?

First, I treated the patient. Second, I reminded myself that the resident's attack on me was not personal. Third, I talked with the resident after he had calmed down.

I explained to him that he was not obligated to treat anyone who refused his sincere efforts to administer care. I also told him that unless he planned to treat only black patients, he could again be confronted by a prejudiced patient who refused his services or, at best, only tolerated his efforts out of necessity. Recognition of equality is not granted simultaneously with the M.D. degree, and all physicians must learn to deal with prejudice, especially if it interferes with the delivery of health care.

Attempting to force a doctor to care for a patient who refuses his services is a disservice to both patient and doctor.

Commentary

In this critical incident a white patient refuses treatment from a black physician. The incident is important not just because of the refusal, but also because the patient goes beyond this to actually insult the doctor.

I would like to discuss not only the specific questions raised by the contributor but the form in which this case is presented by him. It seems to me that this is a rather inadequate presentation—inadequate because it is incomplete and, to my mind, indicates that the contributor is somewhat biased himself. He calls the physician "a black man" without giving any idea as to his age. This is important since we are asked to comment on his behavior, which may be attributable to the immaturity of youth. The contributor also says that the "black man" was from a small town. Is he implying that this doctor lacked something that large cities bring to a physician's ability to deal with difficult patients? He furthermore insinuates that the doctor in question was racially isolated. Nowhere is there any indication that racial tensions in that hospital had received any attention in order to defuse potential explosions such as this one.

The contributor's discussion is simplistic and paternalistic. It is simplistic when he states the obvious that the first order of business is treating the patient. Of course, that comes first when the patient is physically present and suffering. It is very paternalistic when he states that he then "explained" to his black colleague that "he is not obligated . . . etc." Every black physician knows all that this doctor "explained."

I strongly disagree with the handling of this case by the contributor because there is no evidence of true friendliness toward his black colleague who had been so grossly insulted. He simply preached to him, and I feel he added further insult to injury by telling a black doctor that "all physicians must learn to deal with prejudice." This is so grossly paternalistic that I seriously question the white physician's judgment.

The first question in the discussion, namely, "How does one deal with prejudice in medicine?" is never answered. Instead we are given a crisis intervention after the fact as if this were an acceptable response to the question.

The incident has certainly a broad theoretical context, with ethical, social, psychological, political, administrative, and religious perspectives. If we are ever to prevent, or at least reduce, racial clashes in our society, we should make a serious attempt at educating the racists as to the evil consequences of their ways. In this case, once the acute episode was over and the contributor "sat with the patient until he was comfortable," he should have "explained" to his patient that racial insults have no place in a hospital, or anywhere else for that matter, and that it would be best if he—the patient—made a goodwill effort to change. He should also have been told that there could be another emergency situation in which only a black doctor would be available to treat him. Failure to have done this only reinforces negative racist behavior. It also fails to address one of our greatest needs, which is to reduce the isolation and smoldering anger of our minority physicians by failing to support them actively in educating the aggressors in our society.

Jorge Prieto, M.D.
Chairman, Department of Family Practice
Cook County Hospital
Chicago, Illinois

Commentary

This vignette raises, as it was intended to, some very thorny issues, especially the understanding and "contract" between a doctor and his patient, between the patient and the doctor toward whom the patient has strong negative feelings, and the obligations of a hospital toward its residents and trainees. The patient in this situation refuses treatment, demanding it from a white rather than a black doctor. Refusal of treatment is, of course, a patient's prerogative, but under emergency circumstances should a "racially suitable" doctor rush into the breach? I think as a practice, it is very unwise. Although the private physician was there, fortunately, to take over the patient's management in the acute situation, it seems important for the private physician and the patient to draw up an explicit contract for emergency care when the patient is less acutely ill. Unless the private physician can guarantee his availability under all circumstances, an explicit agreement for the patient to accept care from the available physician should be made, with the proviso that if the patient refuses the available treatment (including the available physician), the private physician has no obligation to provide alternate or ongoing care. This patient needs limits to his impossible demands, and unless he is willing to accept such limits (or is rich enough to "own" his own physician for full-time availability), he may find himself forced to receive marginal or no care. All patients must to some extent deal with the reality that they cannot totally control their own health care, which involves some trust, bargaining, and compromise with their own physicians. This patient should be no exception, and the private physician should, I believe, confront the patient with his own behavior, which is both destructive and self-destructive. Obviously, this confrontation should occur when the patient has recovered somewhat from his acute illness.

The issue about the resident feeling "out of place" in the urban center, and then becoming angry when insulted, raises several other issues. Obviously, the resident needs some help in seeing that this is the patient's problem, and not his own, and that an angry response is probably going to help no one in this situation. At the same time, some of this anger is justified, including anger at the hospital and residency program, which did not either warn him or support him in this situation. The private physician, by his behavior, has confirmed the resident's belief that he (the resident) is seen as inferior to a white physician. The hospital and residency program should make clear ahead of time its stance regarding the circumstances of a potentially demanding or difficult patient rejecting a specific resident physician's care. For example, if a hospital accepts a resident for training, is the resident informed of the authority of the private physician to remove him from the case? What are the criteria for this? How are the resident's feelings and lowered self-esteem to be dealt with?

Ultimately, in this age of finite limits on medical resources and escalating costs, the question must be addressed: Is the customer always right? In this situation, the customer and the system are wrong. Should the patient persist in his unreasonable demands and the hospital and private physician acceed to them, then the patient, private physician, and hospital will be participating in their mutual demise.

Hugh James Lurie, M.D.
Clinical Professor of Psychiatry and Behavioral Sciences
University of Washington School of Medicine
Seattle, Washington

23 / Consenting Adults
Homosexual Behavior in the Hospital

Background

On August 28, I admitted Mr. A., a 46-year-old white male, to the hospital because of substernal chest pain and to rule out a myocardial infarction. He had been seen in the office on two occasions earlier in the week and at that time the chest pain was not relieved by antacids. The electrocardiogram showed some slight changes, so he was admitted to the hospital telemetry floor. The patient was exactly my age and had been a personal friend and church vestryman with me during the 15 years I had known him. I felt very anxious to have to admit someone so close to me in age to the hospital with this diagnosis. Following the admission he was seen by a cardiologist, who concurred that he could have coronary artery disease and advised further workup. Just when this was about to be undertaken, his cardiac enzymes returned and they showed elevation of his MB band. His EKG remained stable and it was our feeling that he had suffered a subendocardial myocardial infarction. We then decided to slow down in our workup and to monitor him closely over the next weekend, which happened to be a three-day Labor Day weekend.

The Incident

Mr. A. had been married for 18 years and was a landscape architect. He and his wife had one child, 14 years of age, and his wife worked as a schoolteacher. After being in the hospital for three days the patient was entirely asymptomatic and the small dose of Inderal that he was on made him feel very comfortable. He was riding all over the ward in a wheelchair and generally was very anxious to be discharged from the hospital. With the realization that not much was going to be done over the Labor Day weekend, I decided to make him less agitated. It was beautiful weather and I felt that he could go outside in a wheelchair with appropriate guests, such as his wife.

Later that Saturday evening when I was at a high school football game, I was paged on my "beeper." The telephone to receive this call was in the end zone and with the roar of the crowd it was very hard to hear the nurse at the other end of the line. She told me something about Mr. A. being sent back up to his room by the hospital police because of "necking" on the hospital grounds. I assumed this was with his wife. As I was anxious to get back to the football game, I did not go into much extensive detail with the nurse.

On Sunday morning when I made rounds, I found that this "petting" had taken place on the hospital grounds with a male lover. The nursing staff was much incensed toward me, and I felt in a very awkward position. They then told me that Mr. A. had had male companions in his room during the previous five days of hospitalization. They had been shocked and had felt uneasy about relating these events to me until now.

I went in to see Mr. A. that morning with very great reluctance. It was extremely difficult to talk to him about his bisexuality and homosexuality since I had known him for such an extended length of time without ever going into a discussion like this. I had some inkling about his homosexuality in that he had had venereal warts about his rectum and mouth six months previously. He had chosen to see a dermatologist rather than come to me, and I had received this information from the dermatologist's referral letter. I was very determined in my discussion with him that this homosexuality would not recur on the hospital lawn during the remainder of his hospitalization, and I told him that he would be unable to go outside except in the company of his wife. I then contacted Mrs. A. while I was in the room with him to see if she would come to the hospital that afternoon and take him outside in the sunshine. She agreed to do that and this seemed to relieve Mr. A., as he was going hospital "stir crazy." After leaving the room I then went to the nursing station and recontacted Mrs. A. to see if she had any inkling about her husband's homosexuality. She did but was not very willing to talk about it.

During the remainder of Mr. A.'s hospitalization of four days, he became much less agitated and easier to handle. He still continued to have male companionship in his room, but there was no exhibitionism out in the hall or in visiting rooms. The nursing staff had much difficulty in handling their antihomosexual feelings, although one nurse who had previously had a homosexual husband could relate very well to Mr. A. They had long discussions and this relationship was very helpful in his adjustment to the hospital. A week-and-a-half after admission, he was transferred to another hospital and coronary angiography was performed, which showed complete obstruction of his right coronary artery. He was not felt to be a surgical candidate and so he was discharged home.

Since then I have followed him in the office and we have had many frank discussions about homosexuality and his desire to stop living this double life. He seems relieved to have a friend who knows about this. I have referred him to our common minister and to several psychiatrists. I have also had a meeting with his wife. She has known about the homosexuality since before their marriage in 1962. She is heterosexual. They shared in intercourse about one time per month throughout their marriage. She now finds her husband repulsive. There has been no intercourse since the heart attack. She has decided to get a divorce and start life anew. I advised her to at least put this off until four months after his myocardial infarction, and she agreed to do this. She states she is in no hurry to remarry.

Discussion

I found this to be exceedingly difficult, but interesting and challenging to me. It was my first outright exposure to homosexuality involving someone to whom I was extremely close. Mr. A. had a very serious condition that could have ended terminally. I certainly could not sidestep this homosexual issue and ignore it. It caused a lot of anxiety in me, and my discussion with him on homosexuality was very difficult for me.

I am extremely gratified by the outcome of all this tension, as Mr. and Mrs. A. are still good friends of mine and seem very pleased by the interest that I have taken in the case. With issues regarding sexuality coming to the forefront in recent years, this sort of incident is going to become more common. I think the only way to handle it is to attack it head-on and don't duck it. I had great fears that Mr. A. would sign himself out of the hospital when I talked to him about homosexuality, and I did not want this to happen. It required a lot of listening to the ventilation of his pent-up anxieties. This was a great learning experience for me and I am sure will allow me to be a more understanding physician in the future.

Commentary

The physician in this incident raises no questions himself but highlights the issue of the current changing attitudes toward sexuality. To be sure, the acceptance of varying sexual orientations is more prevalent at the present time. With this acceptance, issues promoted by these orientations will more likely find their way into the family physician's office or other health care facilities. The physician must be prepared to deal with these issues and, in so doing, must have a good understanding of the problems. This should include knowledge about all sexual orientations as well as some understanding of the physician's own feelings about them. The physician's feelings that must be understood range from his or her moral attitudes to his or her own conflicts in the area of sexuality. This speaks, of course, for the inclusion of a study of sexuality in medical school curriculum and in residency training.

Beyond this, the physician should be prepared to assist other personnel such as receptionists, nurses, hospital aides, and technicians in handling aspects of these problems from a perspective of understanding and care-giving. This of course implies that the physician must in some measure be a consultant in the problems of sexuality. He must be able to listen to the concerns and conflicts of his associates and assist them in finding ways of dealing with their patients' problems as well as their own feelings. It is an area which cannot be simply left to the fortuitous chance that one of the nurses or other personnel will be intuitive or understanding about sexual aberration.

Although the sexual problem is a remarkably important aspect of this incident, it seems that a serious underlying problem has been ignored by the physician. This, of course, is the interconnection between the life-threatening events experienced by this patient and his current dramatic change in be-havior. Although his bisexuality had been present for an extended period, it is only at this time that he chose to display it so openly and with such poor judgment. In so doing, the patient alienated hospital staff, compromised his relationship to his physician friend, and precipitated the potential divorce from his wife. It is not uncommon within the experience of death-dealing disorders that the ensuing depression causes an individual to retreat from his or her usual supports. Either the person rejects those around him or his irritable, depressed behavior causes others to reject him. Often at the basis of this behavior is tremendous fear and anger at the unknown and what fate has produced.

Thus, discussing the bisexuality alone would be helpful but not thorough. Efforts at talking about the patient's concerns over his heart and his anxiety about the changes this will produce are essential. This will potentially con-front his feelings of loss, inadequacy, and intense anger. Discussing the patient's emotional reactions to his physical illness seems very appropriate for the family physician to do. If the patient continues to display his sexual behavior with poor judgment or is distressed by his sexual behavior, a referral to a psychiatrist would be appropriate.

The wife in this incident bears some consideration. She apparently knew about her husband's bisexuality for several years and had made an adjust-ment. At this time of crisis and with her husband's indiscreet exposure of his problem, she, out of embarrassment and anger, decided that she had had enough. Her decision is as impulsive as his display of his bisexual problem. With a potential for her guilt over deserting him at a time when he has serious physical problems, she might be advised to wait not only for him but for herself. She may have misgivings at a later time about giving up a marriage in which she had made an adjustment for so many years. Marital counseling may be indicated.

Nothing has been mentioned about the 14-year-old. Interestingly, the sex of this child was left out of the history. The relevance of this to the effect of the father's open homosexuality would be significant. The family physician should obviously be concerned about the impact on the child of the incident and the decision to divorce. The likelihood that the child was also aware of the father's behavior prior to the hospitalization must be explored to determine what conflicts this might have produced. The decision by the mother to divorce could bring the child into conflict with her. The adolescent is in a sensitive developmental period and would be seriously affected by a crisis of this dimension.

The important lesson to be learned from an incident such as this is not to be misled by surface manifestations which lead away from more critical problems. Here the issue of the patient's anger, sense of inadequacy, and need to avoid confrontation over his serious illness all were masked by his sexual acting-out. The situation impacts on his wife and child, producing a further crisis. Left unattended, these problems could lead to serious depression and family pathology at a later time.

Joel P. Zrull, M.D.
Professor and Chairman, Department of Psychiatry
Medical College of Ohio at Toledo
Toledo, Ohio

Commentary

This case illustrates the complex and difficult types of situations family physicians can experience and the anxiety these situations can produce. It also illustrates how family physicians must characteristically deal with their patients on both the physical and psychological levels.

It is not hard to understand this physician's anxiety. He states he felt initially anxious when he admitted a long-term friend to the hospital with a diagnosis of coronary artery disease, presumably because it reminded him that people of his age group are susceptible to this disease. In addition to this, he had to confront the subject of homosexuality, perhaps on a more direct and personal level than he ever had to before. And on top of this, he had to deal with a hospital ward staff which was not tolerating the situation well.

Let us examine this physician's method of handling the situation. In spite of his anxiety, he chose a direct approach to the problem, to "attack it head-on and don't duck it." He spoke directly to both the patient and to his wife about the patient's homosexuality. As a first step, the patient was told that the acting out of his homosexual orientation must not take place on hospital grounds. Then, the physician had long discussions with the patient. The patient also had talks with the nurse who had previously had a homosexual husband. After the hospitalization, the physician had follow-up discussions with both the patient and his wife regarding the future direction of their lives.

Three issues relevant to family physicians are raised by this case. The first involves dealing with variant social behaviors and their social manifestations in medical practice. I believe this physician was correct in strongly discouraging the acting-out of his patient's homosexuality in the hospital, since this was likely to and did produce very real negative social consequences, that is, the negative reactions of the ward staff and the patient's wife. However, the patient should be allowed to express any personal thoughts or desires to the physician privately. This physician should be commended for the direct and open approach he took toward the patient, as I believe it was the most beneficial avenue. The chances of survival for the patient's marriage are probably limited, however. Homosexuals who are strongly motivated to live as heterosexuals, particularly if they are bisexual, can often be helped in doing this by counseling or psychotherapy. I suspect this physician's follow-up discussions concerning the patient's desire to stop living a double life and his urging his wife to wait a period before seeking a divorce will give the marriage its full option to go in either direction.

It should be mentioned that one might object on moral grounds to the physician's speaking to the wife about her husband's homosexuality without consulting the patient first. If the patient had been keeping his homosexuality a secret from his wife, discussing it with her might have been interpreted as a breach of patient confidentiality and may have had adverse consequences for his therapeutic relationship with the family unit. However, since in this case the wife did, in fact, have prior knowledge about her husband's sexual preference, no harm was done.

The second issue is the method this physician used to cope with his anxiety over this situation. In spite of the fact that it increased his initial discomfort, he chose confrontation. It worked for him, and he looks back on the situation as a challenge and a positive learning experience. I suspect, however, that not all physicians would be capable of the same approach. A physician who feels uncomfortable with the subject of homosexuality or who doesn't feel he has the time to deal with the problem in a similar fashion should probably refer these patients to a physician who has the time and a different perspective on the subject.

The third issue, which perhaps is incidental, has to do with the ethical and psychological aspects of a physician treating his close friends. One could argue that the physician should not have treated his particular friend because of his previous close relationship with him. One could also argue that his anxiety over the situation could lead him to be nonobjective in his treatment and have adverse effects on the therapy he gives. After much psychological struggling, it worked for this physician. But again, it might not have for every physician.

Richard I. Haddy, M.D.
Private Practice
Mid-Michigan Family Medical Center
Grand Ledge, Michigan

Suggested Reading

Cadoret, R. J., & King, L. J. *Psychiatry in primary care*. St. Louis: Mosby, 1974.

24 / "Let Them Rant and Rave"
The Noncompliant, Demanding Patient

Background

This elderly, female patient, wife of a retired V.I.P. in the community, dwells in past glories. She has a gross Parkinsonian tremor with expressionless facies, but denies her difficulty. She refuses to take appropriate medication, keeps wanting to try inappropriate medication (such as B_{12} injections), and continually seeks physicians who will agree with her own theories as to what is wrong with her. She complains to her family and friends continually without heeding their advice, and in general alienates all the people she knows and meets, then wonders why nobody listens to her.

The Incident

Each time this patient pays an office visit it is a critical incident. The best way of defusing the incident is to shut up. Gradually, over a period of a half-hour, she will tire of telling you what is wrong with your office help, what is wrong with yourself, and the tone of her words begins to take the form of a plea, asking what she can do to help herself. At this time you may start to get a word in edgewise and, if you are firm, you might sell her on the need of taking anti-Parkinsonian medication. Finally, she will become passive and run out of words and, feeling the passage of time, will take her leave. You can rest assured that by the time she reaches home she will have forgotten her passiveness, will refuse to take her medication, and will begin an argument with whoever is next to cross her path.

Discussion

I think this type of patient will forever be a problem. My experience tells me that these people are problems even to psychiatrists. As far as I know, the best advice, when they are encountered, is to keep quiet, shrug your shoulders, and let them rant and rave.

Commentary

The patient noted in this critical incident, though difficult to manage, is not impossible to deal with given a reasonable understanding of her unconscious and conscious motives as they pertain to her chronic illness and its relationship to her past history and present family structure. Parkinson's disease is an illness that would have numerous ramifications to this formerly active wife of a retired V.I.P. She is probably confronted with a fixed facial expression, a slow and decreased motor activity, and a probable tremor, all of which can be exacerbated and considerably worsened by emotional or psychological factors such as unhappiness, anxiety, and depression. This older woman, who formerly had an important role in society as she saw it and as others viewed her, now has been reduced to an individual who probably feels self-pity as a result of a poor body image and feels bitter and angry toward an affliction over which she has little if any control. Her independence in the past now will result in dependence on other individuals, such as physicians and other health care team members. This dependence would be very difficult for her to accept because of her active social past.

Some physicians would classify this patient into the category of the "entitled demander." The entitled demander is one who attempts to belittle and intimidate the physician while attempting to instill guilt for his lack of success in managing the problem. She may see the same physician repeatedly, or when unhappy or dissatisfied with his results, she may attempt to see numerous other physicians as well. This type of patient is extremely dependent upon the physician, though she does not recognize this and demonstrates instead hostility and anger. Her real fear is, in fact, fear of abandonment. The involved physician, however, is of course distraught by his lack of success, and of course worried that this patient may be harmful to his reputation as well as to his psyche. The physician may soon, on account of ineffective management, begin to question his own competence. This type of patient, if not recognized for what she is, results in a distressing problem that drains the energies of those of us who have the best intentions.

This patient is also used to giving advice rather than accepting advice, and now must be educated and dealt with in a fashion that will allow her to become a respected partner in the management of her illness. By seeing this patient on a very regular basis, probably weekly at first, the physician may slowly develop rapport and a better understanding of the patient's needs. During this process, the patient can be educated completely about the disease and how it can be partially or completely controlled by medication so that relative ly normal function can be returned.

It is important to note that this patient, because of her illness and change of lifestyle, may have become depressed. By recognizing these possibilities and by attempting to deal with them as well, a more complete picture of the total management of this patient would evolve. Patient education may include a description of the types of medications and how they may help, a time frame for possible results associated with drug manipulation, and also an introduc tion to other patients with the same condition who have been helped. This final suggestion may aid the patient in accepting treatment, regular visits, and help that she had initially rejected. The most recent literature now supports an increased frequency of dementia and Alzheimer-like changes than had previously been thought to be associated with this particular condition (Boller & Mizutani, 1980; Halsim & Mathiesen, 1979). Though these changes prob ably occur fairly late in the disease, awareness of their possible occurrence is important and may influence one's overall management.

Are these patients problems to psychiatrists? This type of patient would, of course, be a problem to any physician who does not attempt to assess the patient in the context of past history as well as present family structure as thoroughly as possible. This patient can become a partner in her own care by helping to develop a care plan with her physician that would contribute to her recovery. She may become involved with relatives who, given a fresh approach, may be willing to contribute some time and effort in the rehabilita tion of this patient.

What about the question of the B_{12} injection and whether or not it is appropriate? Vogel and Goodwin have quoted Wolfe as defining the placebo response as "any effect attributable to a pill, potion, or procedure, but not to its pharmaco-dynamic or specific properties" (1980). Recent studies have shown that deception is not a requirement for the effective use of a placebo, and even when patients are advised that they are receiving substances which have no specific effect on their symptoms, a substantial number will still respond to this treatment. When a diagnosis is known and established, it is not unreasonable to use a placebo in conjunction with other effective drugs or modes of therapy if, in fact, the patient can associate the placebo with meaningful results. If the patient requested the injection, it may allow the patient some measure of immediate improvement as well as some gratification in the cooperative management of her own disease with probably little or no harm. So to speak, it may permit the family physician to get his "foot in the door." I believe it is the appropriate application of the placebo, just as the appropriate touch of the physician's hand or his or her listening ear, is an integral part of the "art of medicine" and separates the experienced, wise physician from the graduate medical doctor. The complicated, chronically ill patient may require all of the tools of our trade including placebos for effective management.

There are some broader issues we must consider in the light of this case. Medalie speaks eloquently to the presence of the "hidden patient" or "care-taker" (1978). He notes that in the management of the chronically ill patient, there is frequently a spouse or other closely related individual who is so involved with the patient, and possibly so distraught over the patient's illness, that he may surprise us by presenting to our office with a stress ulcer, extreme depression, or other serious complication if we are not in tune with this possibility. Therefore, an important issue is to consider the other members of the family who have been burdened by this patient's illness and look upon them not only for their help, but possibly to attend to their own personal needs as the situation dictates. By overlooking the "hidden patient," we miss the opportunity for preventive medicine, a key ingredient in the practice of a successful family physician. The social aspects of this particular problem are, of course, the successful return of this person to society so that she may function in an effective manner and contribute in some way rather than to burden us financially. The true "artist" in family medicine looks for a challenge and explores in depth and to the best of his ability all of the ramifications of a patient's illness to aid in restoring the individual, as much as possible, to a useful and meaningful life.

Another and final issue of broad importance is whether or not we have an obligation to help a patient of this type at all. Even though I feel a patient with this particular problem and presentation can be helped, it is a time-consuming process that may tax the busy family practitioner to his own mental and physical limits. Do we have an obligation under these circumstances to attend to this patient or on the contrary are we better off to simply cast them aside and care for other, less demanding individuals? Morally, does the principle of beneficence which refers to acts involving prevention of harm, helping others, removal of harmful conditions, and positive benefiting obli-gate us to pursue the needs of this individual? The physician in the Hippocra-tic Oath is committed to "come only for the good of my patients" and to "prescribe regimen for the good of my patients according to my ability and my judgment and never do harm to anyone" (*Stedman's Medical Dictionary*, 1976, p. 647). In the AMA's code, "The prime objective of the medical profession is to render service to humanity" (American Medical Association, 1949, p. 3), with full respect for the dignity of man. On the other hand, according to the AMA code, "A physician may choose whom he will serve" (American Medical Association, 1949, p. 10). In the final analysis the family physician is a personal physician who practices comprehensive, humanistic, and scientific medicine oriented around an individual in the context of his family. We are the patient's first and often final bridge to a healthy life and whenever possible we must do our best to serve him.

As Sir William Osler wrote in 1899:

> Be careful when you get into practice to cultivate equally well your hearts and your heads. There is a strong feeling abroad among people that we doctors are given over nowadays to science—we care much more for the disease and the scientific aspects of it than for the individual. I would urge upon you to care more particularly for the individual patient than for the special features of the disease. Dealing as we do with poor, suffering humanity, we see the man unmasked or, so to speak, exposed to all the frailties and weaknesses. You have to keep your heart pretty soft and pretty tender not to get too great a contempt for your fellow creatures. The best way to do that is to keep a looking glass in your hearts, and the more carefully you scan your own frailties, the more tender you are for the frailties of your fellow creatures [Osler, 1899, pp. 307–309].

Philip Caravella, M.D.
Director, Family Practice
Riverside Hospital
Toledo, Ohio

References and Suggested Readings

American Medical Association. *Principles of medical ethics of the American Medical Association*. Chicago: Author, 1949.

Beauchamp, T. L., & Childress, J. F. *Principles of biomedical ethics*. New York: Oxford University Press, 1979.

Boller, F., & Mizutani, T. Parkinson's disease, dementia, and Alzheimer's disease: Clinicopathological correlations. *Annals of Neurology*, April 1980, 7(4), 329–335.

Cousins, N. Anatomy of an illness (as perceived by the patient). *Saturday Review*, May 1977.

Freedman, A. *Comprehensive text of psychiatry II* (2nd ed.). Baltimore: Williams & Wilkins, 1975.

Groves, J. Taking care of the hateful patient. *New England Journal of Medicine*, 1978, 298(16), 883–887.

Halsim, A., & Mathiesen, G. Dementia in Parkinson's disease: A neuropathological study. *Neurology*, September 1979, 1208–1209.

Medalie, J. H. The family life cycle and its implications for family practice. *Journal of Family Practice*, 1979, 9(1), 47–56.

Medalie, J. H. *Family medicine: Principles and applications*. Baltimore: Williams & Wilkins, 1978.

Osler, W. Address to the students of the Albany Medical College. *Albany Medical Annals*, 1899, *20*(6), 307–309.

Pickering, G. Therapeutics: Art or science? *Journal of the American Medical Association*, 1979, *242*(7), 649–653.

Stedman, T. L. *Medical Dictionary: A vocabulary of medicine and its allied sciences with pronunciation and derivations* (23rd ed.). Baltimore: Williams and Wilkins, 1976.

Vogel, A., & Goodwin, J. The therapeutics of placebo. *American Family Physician*, 1980, *22*(1), 105.

Commentary

This brief incident poignantly illustrates a situation that should be familiar to any physician: despite his best efforts and intentions, this doctor has become frustrated with his patient. The extent of his frustration is clearly illustrated in the language that he uses to describe her behavior: she "dwells," she "denies," she "refuses," she "keeps wanting," she "continually seeks," she "complains," she "alienates," and she "wonders." In short, this patient has clearly "gotten under the skin" of the physician. This is succinctly summarized by his remarkable statement that "every time she pays an office visit it is a critical incident." The poignancy of this statement is found in its universality: all of us in the helping professions have encountered clients who have elicited strong negative reactions on our parts. Reading this incident I can experience the physician's feelings of anxious anticipation and even dread that would precede walking into the examination room in which she was waiting. The danger of a situation such as this is that it tends to feed on itself: once a tear in the doctor–patient relationship has started, it can create a vicious circle of physician frustration causing patient alienation and vice versa. At its worst, it can interfere with the well-being of the patient, the *sine qua non* of medical care. In addition, it can take its emotional toll of the physician and can be implicated in what is now being called "burnout" (Edelwich & Brodsky, 1980).

Traditionally the situation described in this incident would fit into the rubric of "the problem patient." The stereotype of the "problem patient" would most likely be the demanding, noncompliant patient who presents with vague, functional complaints and most likely would have psychiatric or other emotional difficulties (Malcolm, Foster, & Smith, 1977). These are the patients who are given the unfortunate appellations of "crock" or "turkey." While the patient involved in this critical incident does not fit the stereotype because she has organic pathology, Malcolm et al. (1977) also make the point that the most important feature of "the problem patient" is that he or she "creates difficulties in the process of developing and maintaining a normative physician–patient relationship" (Malcolm et al., 1977, p. 61). There is no doubt that the patient in question creates such difficulties.

The implication of this traditional line of thinking relevant to the "problem patient" is that there is something about the patient which causes the doctor to become frustrated or depressed. This view of seeing the problem as residing primarily or solely in the patient has rightfully been challenged. It has become clear that this type of disruptive, emotionally charged doctor–patient relationship is the result of an interaction between the doctor and the patient. In the words of Kaywin (1973), it reflects an "illness of interaction," not just the personality and/or behavior of the patient. This would explain why the same patient may be problematic to one physician but not to another.

To say that troubled physician–patient relationships are the result of an interaction between the two participants does not mean that patients are uniformly easy or pleasant to deal with. Rather, some patients might have a greater likelihood of being involved in troubled relationships. However, in such instances, the physician must be seen as having the power and responsibility to keep the relationship from deteriorating.

Steiger and Hirsch (1965) have presented a thoughtful analysis of the problematic doctor–patient relationship from the interactionist perspective. They view the interaction between physician and patient as being comprised of a series of "offers" by the patient and "responses" by the physician. They described 10 types of patients that are likely to present offers which have a likelihood of leading to trouble if they are not countered by appropriate physician responses. The 10 types of patients are as follows: the multiple complainer, the silent or uninformative patient, the verbose or tangential talker, the masochistic patient, the patient who presents a "red-herring disease," the hysterical or dissociated patient, the psychotic patient, the severely depressed patient, the hostile patient, and the arrogant or critical patient. Of course, this list could be expanded.

Presumably, any troublesome patient offer can be met with either adaptive of maladaptive physician responses. An adaptive response would be one which "defuses" the situation, avoiding a deterioration in the doctor–patient relationship. A maladaptive response would be one which further compounds the situation. Malcolm et al. (1977) also present nine physician attitudes and behaviors that can lead to maladaptive responses: not admitting imperfection, trying to make our patients live up to our standards, frustration or rejection, overidentification with the patient, intellectualization and the use of professional terminology, treatment of the manifest complaint, treatment of the chance objective finding, premature reassurance and advice giving, and avoidance of the sexual areas of the patient's life. This list could also be expanded.

What makes a physician take the bait of the patient and respond maladaptively? That is a question that does not seem to have received much attention. Malcolm et al. (1977) found that some physicians reported encountering a number of problem patients that was disproportionately high in comparison to other physicians. In fact, some reported having seen thousands of problem patients. Thus, just as there are patients who have a greater likelihood of being involved in problematic relationships with doctors, some physicians are also more likely to be involved in troubled relationships with patients.

I do not wish to imply that the physician in this incident is a "problem doctor." That brings up a very important point: any physician, given the wrong patient at the wrong time, can find him- or herself involved in a problematic relationship. One reason for this is that we are subject to emotions that are beyond our control. Some psychotherapists refer to this phenomenon as "countertransference." Our past histories, current needs, and emotional states can interfere with our judgments. Sometimes the "chemistry" between the doctor and the patient is such that it elicits a strong reaction. Perhaps the patient reminds the physician of an important figure in his or her life. Or perhaps the patient reminds him or her of a past success or failure. Furthermore, even if no such similarity exists, at certain times we are more vulnerable to failure or the threat of failure—such as when one has a sense of failure about another case or when one has even minor problems in other areas of life, for example, problems with children, in-laws, or with the Chief of Staff. Again, I would like to stress that we are all subject to such vulnerabilities.

Let me return to the incident. What should this physician do now that he finds himself in this situation? The first thing is to try to ascertain exactly what is so frustrating about this woman. As Steiger (1967) points out, awareness is the key. The physician should do some soul searching to figure out just what about the patient's personality and behavior bothers him. Perhaps more important, he should then try to decide why it bothers him so much. Next, he should try to understand how his attitudes and behaviors contribute to the problem. He might review the list of Steiger and Hirsch that I have cited above. In addition, he should ask himself whether his expectations differ from hers. His priority (with justification) has been compliance. On the other hand, the priority of this lonely, unloved old woman might be to have a sympathetic listener. Along these lines, it could be that she is not nearly as dissatisfied with him as he believes and the reduction in tension that she probably receives from unloading her problems on him is most likely in itself therapeutic. The physician should keep in mind that her psychosocial problems are interfering with her physical problems and that improvement in the latter might well depend on improvement in the former. This will take time and patience. He should also consider formalizing a treatment contract with this patient. The rationale behind this would be to try to clarify her role in the treatment process.

The physician clearly seems frustrated at the amount of his time that this woman consumes with such little observable result. Perhaps redefining the problem, as I just did above, might help him to be more patient. Another thing that would attenuate the problem of how much time she demands is to rely more on the team approach, for instance, let her spend time talking to a nurse or to other office staff members. In addition, the doctor might see what supports in the community might help to lighten his load, for example, clergymen or a social service agency. Finally, referral to a social worker, psychologist, or psychiatrist might be considered.

Now that I have addressed what this physician can do once he has found himself in this situation, I would like to examine what can be done in general to prevent this situation from occurring. First, it is altogether imperative that physicians pay attention to their emotional reactions to patients. Once they find themselves reacting strongly to a patient, they should examine their reaction by asking questions similar to those I have described above. In so doing, it would be most helpful to discuss the patient and one's reaction to the patient with another person. The sooner that one can gain insight into the origins of the problem, the sooner one can defuse the situation. Again, reliance on the team approach can also help to prevent problematic doctor–patient relationships from building. The more the patient can complain to another member of the health care team, the less the burden placed on the doctor. Enlisting the use of social workers, psychologists, and psychiatrists can also be beneficial, especially if it is done early enough. One of the biggest problems encountered in referrals to one of these specialists is that it is often not done early enough. If the physician waits until a major problem has developed before referral, there is less chance that effective intervention will take place.

Kenneth P. Kushner, Ph.D.
Clinical Assistant Professor, Department of Family Medicine
Medical College of Ohio at Toledo
Toledo, Ohio

References

Edelwich, H. J., & Brodsky, A. Burnout: Stage of disillusionment in the helping profession. New York: Human Sciences Press, 1980.

Kaywin, P. R. Non-Thanksgiving turkey. New England Journal of Medicine, 1973, 289, 1257.

Malcolm, R., Foster, H. K., & Smith, C. The problem patient as perceived by family physicians. The Journal of Family Practice, 1977, 5(3), 361–364.

Steiger, W. A. Managing difficult patients. Psychosomatics, 1967, 8, 305–308.

Steiger, W. A., & Hirsch, H. The difficult patient in everyday medical practice. Medical Clinics of North America, 1965, 49, 1449–1465.

25 / Ease the Pain
Abuse of Medication

Background
A 30-year-old Puerto Rican female had been referred to our office from the emergency room. I was a third-year family practice resident and assumed her care. Over a one-week period she continued to complain of pleuritic chest pain and severe left lower quadrant pain unresponsive to one grain of codeine every four hours. She gave a complicated past medical history consisting of two caesarian deliveries and three episodes of pulmonary thromboembolism, the last occurring seven years prior to her present illness. She stated this last event necessitated an inferior vena caval plication with an incidental bilateral tubal ligation. She had also suffered a bimalleolar fracture of her right leg several years previously with resultant chronic calf pain and stated that she was allergic to Percodan, aspirin, Talwin, and Tigan.

An extensive outpatient workup, consisting of chest and abdominal films, arterial blood gases, pelvic ultrasound, gynecology consult, hematology and chemistry studies, and serum pregnancy tests, was unremarkable. Her physical exam, with particular attention to her abdomen, lungs, and extremities, was also within normal limits.

The Incident
At 6:30 A.M. I received a call from the emergency room stating the patient was there again complaining of severe abdominal and chest pain and gave an

184

added history of syncope, hemoptysis, and fever to 102°. She was admitted with a diagnosis of possible pulmonary thromboembolism.

The ensuing seven days of the patient's hospitalization were marked both by her frequent demands for pain medication in increasing amounts and a thorough negative medical and surgical workup, including electrocardiogram, ventilation-perfusion scan, contrast gastrointestinal and urographic studies, and surgical consultation. Her pain did not improve with empiric antiinflammatory and anticoagulant trial. In fact, at one point she was requiring 10 mg of intravenous morphine every three hours (as she was not a candidate for intramuscular medication while on heparin) despite her five foot, 90-pound frame.

The hemoptysis and temperature elevation were never confirmed while under observation. Her relationship with the nursing personnel was one of constant demands, threats, and importuning. Because of such behavior, the nursing staff conveyed their apprehension to the on-call house staff, who in general, complied by administering narcotic medication.

I felt extremely uncomfortable in dealing with this patient. From the first visit I had attempted to obtain her previous medical records, which she said were forthcoming. However, she later informed me that they were being mailed to her home address because she did not trust hospital medical record departments. Because of her extensive knowledge and familiarity with medical terminology, I was highly suspicious of secondary gain, supported by her list of drug allergies.

During her hospitalization I informed the patient that I had not been able to determine the cause of her pain, and that because of its intensity I felt it necessary to obtain a psychiatric consultation which was an integral part of a complete diagnostic evaluation. She adamantly refused this, saying that she had had an unpleasant experience in the past with psychiatrists and didn't wish to repeat this. She also denied any personal problems or past history of excessive narcotic usage.

I was finally able to contact her previous physician, who stated that he had been the surgical consultant and therefore was not aware of what means had been used to confirm her previous bouts with emboli. Also, he stated that he performed the tubal ligation and an elective, incidental plication procedure on the advice of her medical doctors. He recalled a lengthy hospital stay for her fracture, with excessive narcotic usage.

During the patient's evaluation and empiric trial of medication, I felt reluctant to confront her with my concerns until I had more confidently ruled out serious organic pathology. When I finally did so, she tearfully proclaimed that I was the only one who had understood her and now I was abandoning her. I reiterated my concern for her as a patient but also told her that her behavior was frustrating my efforts to complete her care. She then agreed to be observed off all medications, but left against medical advice a few hours later. The entire experience left me feeling frustrated, defeated, and as if I had indeed not been able to treat her true illness.

Discussion

This case was particularly disturbing to me because, as a family physician, I pride myself with caring for the entire patient. I feel as if my efforts to attend her emotional needs were sabotaged by the patient herself, and that I was unwillingly forced to pursue a mega-workup against my better judgement.

Should I have confronted this patient earlier with the lack of objective evidence for physical disease and her excessive use of narcotics? Should I have been more forceful in requiring an investigation of her emotional health? How could I more tactfully have offered detoxification and rehabilitation for a substance abuser who was obviously an experienced performer? How can a physician more effectively utilize nursing personnel involved with a demanding and difficult patient to avoid the resultant dilemma: the doctor versus the nurse with the patient manipulating their respective behaviors?

Commentary

Ideally, the family physician should have considered from the original history that a central issue in this case was abuse of pain medications. A 30-year-old person with (1) a history of pain-related problems, (2) current chest and abdominal pain, (3) a normal physical exam, (4) lack of relief from a high-dose codeine regimen, and (5) allergies to nonnarcotics should be considered to have a problem of substance abuse, with or without other medical problems. This should not preclude the appropriate diagnostic procedures that were carried out as an outpatient. The early inclusion of pain *per se* and pain medication use as "problems" from the physician's viewpoint can assist in patient management. This must be discussed straightforwardly with the patient.

Investigation of the patient's "emotional health" should consist of the family physician's own adequate understanding of her context: family, occupation, living circumstances, and current stresses. Unless there is evidence of a psychiatric disorder, which is not presented in this case history, referral is inappropriate. Management of substance abuse must begin with candid discussion of the problem, with insistence that its treatment is part of the regimen. On the other hand, diagnostic measures and management must also be aimed at any underlying pathology that can be identified. Detoxification and rehabilitation are crucial to this patient's treatment, but, like any behavioral modification, they require motivation on the patient's part. The physician must care, educate, and offer the expertise of himself and others; then the patient must accept or refuse his or her recommendations.

The physician, medical social worker (or other behavioral science resource person), nursing staff, and family can all be involved in contracting with the patient to manage difficult illness behavior. Communication and consistent responses are essential. The patient must continually be made aware that the medical team will try to help her, and the medical team must be able to demand behavior that is consonant with *their* well-being as persons with full jobs to perform.

My own disagreement with the handling of the final incident is the attempt to make a contract with the patient that she be observed off all medications. She was informed of the concerns about her substance abuse as an alternative to having "serious organic pathology" after the latter had been "ruled out." This was accompanied by a confrontation of her behavior that was creating a problem for the health professionals. All together, the message had to have been: "The jig's up. You're going cold turkey." In addition to the punitive nature of the plan, it would seem to have been an ultimatum that would exclude the patient's participation in the decisions. A frequent response to that loss of control is to show the system who's really the boss by leaving against medical advice.

In family medicine relatively simple measures can usually resolve this type of illness behavior problem. Most are not as severe as this patient, who has both a narcotic addiction and a possible personality disorder. Conjoint management with a psychiatrist would be appropriate *after* the patient had agreed to work on her addiction. Assisting her in life changes that would reduce the need for this way of coping would be central to long-term counseling. From the onset the medical team should be aware that the patient will probably choose not to modify her behavior. Still, they should present the problem and its management in as supportive and optimistic a fashion as possible. The patient must accept responsibility for using or not using available medical expertise. Her awareness of caring and acceptance from those offering to help and her sense of her own control over the decisions and plans will possibly allow her to consider her course of action more rationally.

Vital points are raised by this case:

1.   The biopsychosocial approach to patients in family practice would dictate that their problems, including pleuritic chest pain and LLQ abdominal pain, have to be understood *contextually* by obtaining data about family, occupation, living circumstances, and current stresses in addition to biomedical information about the symptoms and signs.
2.   Comprehensive problem identification in family practice would include specific focus on the use of narcotic pain medications along with other patient problems.
3.   The etiology of patient problems must be assumed by the family physician to have *both* biomedical and psychosocial components, though the proportions will vary.

4.   The "medical model" must be supplemented when necessary by the
     "learning model" in order to understand and treat patients effectively.

The first three points need little elaboration in this case. Little data is
reported about the patient as a person. Indirectly, inferences are made about
her behavior being manipulative and demanding, but we have no information
about her mood, intelligence, thought content or processes, interpersonal
style, or appearance.

The most important feature of this case is the misunderstanding and frustration that occur when the patient's identified problem does not fit the "medical
model." This model assumes that the physician's role is the determination of
the pathology underlying her symptoms and that the effective eradication of
that pathology will cure the patient. The patient turns out to have no causative
pathology underlying her symptoms, so the physician becomes angry about
the energy, time, money, and caring spent looking for it. Her behavior is seen
as deceiving and self-serving for "secondary gain."

An alternative "learning model" could be considered as the physician
quickly becomes aware of the use of potent "pleasure reinforcers" (narcotics),
the history of painful conditions, the past behavior subsequent to previous
illness, and illness behavior in the hospital to obtain medication. Being
symptomatic has a remarkable payoff for some persons, depending upon their
life circumstances: attention from family and friends, care from the physician
and other members of the health care team, avoidance of aversive situations
(possibly work, relationships, anxiety, home, financial stress, or other responsibilities), pleasure of intoxication, and other sick-role benefits.

Family physicians should consider the role of learning, especially in problems of chronic pain, substance abuse, hypochondriasis, depression, and
insomnia. It can be very useful to ask about the circumstances (time and
setting) of the occurrence of the symptoms and the results (what the patient
and others do differently) of the complaint, behavior, or feeling. Often the
problem begins as a typical response to trauma or illness but may persist
because of sick-role reinforcers. It is unnecessary to consider the motivation of
the patient and *blame* them for using these reinforcers for "secondary gain." It
is more appropriate to understand the learning aspects and institute a relearn-
ing process, if necessary. This means enlisting the patient, family, and health
care team in assisting the reinforcement of more healthful behaviors. Specifically, the following rules may be enacted to modify illness behavior: (1) use
medications at effective doses on a *regular* (not PRN) schedule with a plan to
diminish or stop in a prescribed time; (2) praise accomplishments in improved
function, rather than disability; (3) see the patient regularly and briefly with
plans to minimize visits based upon time rather than becoming well; (4)
contract to provide as much support and nurturance as possible without
allowing patient demands that cause resentment and rejection; (5) make

expectations realistic; helping the patient does not require complete etiological understanding or expectation of complete cure.

Richard M. Baker, M.D.
Associate Professor of Family Medicine
University of North Carolina School of Medicine
Chapel Hill, North Carolina

Suggested Readings

Fordyce, W. E. *Behavioral methods for chronic pain and illness*. St. Louis: Mosby, 1976.
Schaefer, H. H., & Martin, P. L. *Behavioral therapy*. New York: McGraw-Hill, 1969.

Commentary

This incident raises a number of interesting, important, and complex issues in the treatment of a difficult patient in an ambiguous situation.

My main concern in the resident's description of this case is the lack of a psychosocial context for the patient's complaints. The background section includes no social or psychological history; the patient is presented as if she were primarily a vehicle for physical symptoms. The author does note that the patient is Puerto Rican, but I am not sure why we are told this since any possible effects and implications are not developed. More complete knowledge of the patient's background might have helped the physician consider a different class of diagnosis from the outset. It also would have been helpful to involve the patient's family since the family can often make valuable contributions to both diagnosis and management, if invited to help. In fact, without this invitation, the physician may set the stage for a later triangulated relationship between the physician, the patient, and the patient's family in which any two of the parties arrange themselves in shifting alliances against the third.

A second major point that this case raises is the fact that the doctor and patient never agreed on a diagnosis. Michael Balint (1964) has written quite persuasively of the necessity for doctor and patient to negotiate a diagnosis together before treatment can proceed as a cooperative venture. In this case, however, the physician does a number of procedures to the patient without ever fully discussing the medical situation with the patient. As a result, the patient becomes a passive spectator while the doctor proceeds as the knowledgeable expert in search of the ultimate lab value (Szasz & Hollender, 1956). Since the patient is not expected to take an active role in the diagnostic process, her attempts to keep certain information from the physician are given little attention. In this kind of hierarchical relationship, a manipulative patient can use her passivity to maintain enough uncertainty to defeat even the best-intentioned workup. Medical care, of course, often takes place in the face of incomplete information, which is anxiety provoking for all concerned. In this case, some of the patient's somatic complaints may well have been related to drug abuse or withdrawal (Berger, 1979; Detzer, Muller & Carlin, 1977), but without a more detailed history, this possibility is unlikely to be considered.

The patient's increasing demands for pain medication and narcotics obviously troubled the third-year resident. I was quite concerned, however, to note the house staff's response to nursing's complaints about the patient. "Constant demands, threats, and importuning" are not FDA approved indications for narcotics, although such behavior is certainly an appropriate trigger for intervention. Medication was apparently given to quiet the nursing staff as much as the patient. This incident could have provided the opportunity for constructive outside consultation to deal with the patient, the nursing staff, and the house staff together in a more coherent, systematic fashion. Although I do not doubt the ability of this demanding patient to fuel staff anxiety and anger, palliative narcotics have expensive and often tragic consequences.

The resident's attempts to get psychiatric consultation were refused—a common situation, particularly with a substance abuser (Dubovsky & Weissberg, 1978). This left the resident in an increasingly difficult situation, namely, what to do if the patient denies the doctor permission to get additional consultation when more information is needed to manage the case properly. There may be occasions when a patient's refusal to allow consultation should lead the attending physician to dismiss the case. This is less likely in the case of refused psychiatric consultation since the refusal will probably not lead to immediate or fatal consequences. If the resident was unwilling to continue treatment without psychiatric consultation, the patient might simply have signed out sooner and used the incident to justify leaving against medical advice. One alternative to direct psychiatric consultation is for the attending physician to use the consultant himself. Although this may limit a consultant's effectiveness, it does allow entry of an uninvolved and expert third party who might offer valuable and timely suggestions. In this case, psychiatric consultation might have raised strong suspicions about the patient's mixed motivations for hospitalization and pain medication. In the absence of "objective information," however, a manipulative patient can often achieve whatever ends he or she desires. As the physician becomes more dependent on the patient's integrity for rational management of the case, his own anxiety and sense of helplessness are likely to increase. This, in turn, may heighten the physician's vulnerability to personal emotional reactions to the patient, which leads to even less rational management.

The physician's reluctance to confront the patient until he "had more confidently ruled out serious organic pathology" suggests the kind of dichotomous "either . . . or" thinking that has been pervasive in this case. As the "organic option" becomes less likely in the face of unremarkable findings, the physician is left in the unenviable position of having to "suddenly" consider a psychological explanation. In the active doctor–passive patient relationship which has been established, it would necessitate a major change in framework to evaluate the possibility that the patient was actively involved in the formation of her symptomatology. Unfortunately, this kind of doctor–patient relationship fails most dramatically when there is much medical uncertainty or when there is a large psychological component in the presenting complaint. It is not surprising, then, that the patient feels upset when the doctor suddenly suggests that the problem may "really" be primarily "psychological."

Ideally, the resident would have taken a more comprehensive approach to his patient beginning from the first office visit. By thinking in terms of a potential "double diagnosis" which includes both organic and psychological factors (and their interaction), the physician and patient might never come to the moment when the patient stalks angrily out of the hospital. Double diagnosis helps to prevent many of the insults that occur to patients as a result of negative workups which lead to the unattractive (and often simplistic) alternative, "You mean it's all in my head?" By the time this resident does confront his patient, she may well assume rejection is forthcoming since she has kept information from him and drug abusers generally do not expect gentle treatment when the abuse is discovered (Detzer et al., 1977; Lipp, 1977). The physician may be feeling a mixture of anger, guilt, and inadequacy both for his potential contribution to this unsatisfying outcome and for his willingness "to pursue a mega-workup against my better judgment." In some cases, the unwary physician may subtly encourage the patient to angrily leave his care thereby allowing the doctor to blame the patient while ignoring his own collusion in the end result (Groves, 1978). Thus the transaction is complete as the resident says (gratefully) "another crock," while the patient turns angrily to mutter, "another heartless quack."

This commentary, of course, is written with all the perspicacity of hindsight. The pressures induced by this kind of case are enormous. The uncertainty of the presenting symptomatology, the difficulty obtaining reliable information, the demanding and manipulative nature of the patient, the patient's ability to mobilize her environment against her—all becloud an already confusing, evocative, and draining situation.

William T. Merkel, Ph.D.
Assistant Professor
Wright State University School of Medicine
Wright State University School of Professional Psychology
Dayton, Ohio

References

Balint, M. *The doctor, his patient and the illness* (2nd ed.). New York: Pitman, 1964.

Berger, P., & Tinkelenberg, J. Medical management of the drug abuser. In A. Freeman, R. Stack, & P. Berger (Eds.), *Psychiatry for the primary care physician*. Baltimore: Williams & Wilkins, 1979.

Detzer, E., Muller, B., & Carlin, A. Identifying and treating the drug-misusing patient. *American Family Physician*, 1977, *16*, 181–186.

Dubovsky, S., & Weissberg, M. *Clinical psychiatry in primary care*. Baltimore: Williams & Wilkins, 1978.

Groves, J. Taking care of the hateful patient. *The New England Journal of Medicine*, 1978, *298*, 883–887.

Lipp, M. *Respectful treatment*. Hagerstown, Md.: Harper & Row, 1977.

Szasz, T., & Hollender, M. H. A contribution to the philosophy of medicine—the basic models of the doctor–patient relationship. *Archives of Internal Medicine*, 1956, *97*, 585–592.

26 / Only If God Allows
Religious Behavior vs. Medical Science

Background

I entered my office pediatric room to greet a new patient family. The mother
was in her late 20s and seemed pleasant and appropriate. A three-and-one-
half-year-old daughter was on the examining table and a one-year-old daughter was on her mother's lap. The appointment was for a pre-nursery school
examination. After taking the usual history, which included a normal pregnancy and delivery, normal development without serious injury, illness, or
operation, I proceeded with the physical exam. Examination was normal
except for resolving bilateral otitis media. When I again asked questions
concerning the ears, this time the mother told me that the patient had an
upper respiratory infection 10 days previously and since then the mother had
noted a decrease of hearing. At this point I discussed with the mother that her
child was in good health other than her otitis media, which should be treated,
and that she was due for boosters of her immunizations which had been given
as a baby.

The Incident

The mother then explained her religious convictions. She stated that she was
an R.N. who used to work in a pediatrician's office. Her husband was a college
graduate civil engineer. Since the patient's initial series of immunizations,
they had a change of religious conviction and did not believe in immunizations. The younger child had not received any. She would accept the written

prescription, but stated that she and her husband would "pray about the matter to see if God would direct us to have the prescription filled and to give the medication to our daughter." She then told me that she was referred to me by a certain member of our medical school faculty who is a friend of theirs. She stated that he had told her that he felt that I would understand their conviction and respect it.

I found myself quite taken aback by her statements. I felt angry and saw myself as being set up by my colleague and used by the patient's mother. In searching for a response to her, the following thoughts ran through my head: (1) show my frustration or anger and tell her that if she didn't want to do things my way, don't come back; (2) enter a philosophical or religious debate to prove that my religious and scientific system was better than hers; (3) keep quiet and try to hide my feelings and hope, with time, to prove that I was right, or to gain trust and bend her to a persuasion that I could work with; (4) call the Child Abuse and Neglect Agency; (5) say what's the use—it's their problem.

In actuality, my response to her was essentially as follows: I discussed with the mother that although I realized that we all have different backgrounds and experiences which result in different beliefs and philosophies, by my training and responsibility I must strongly recommend the immunization program as defined by the state and the medical profession. I continued to tell her that if she chose not to participate, I would ask her to sign a release of responsibility and that she should expect me to continue to encourage her in the future to protect her child against these illnesses. She did not immunize her child and signed the form.

Discussion

I consider myself to have religious convictions and respect the beliefs of others. I also believe in medical science and I feel I practice a system of medicine that is within acceptable scientific and ethical standards. However, this case generated a conflict between my respect of others' beliefs and medical science. I find myself wondering whether I was correct in retaining her as a patient, especially in light of the feelings of anger the situation aroused in me.

A second question this incident raises is how should I deal with the colleague who referred her to me? I assume that one of the reasons he referred her to me is that he knows I am a religious individual. Yet I feel he should have spoken to me about her before sending her over.

Commentary

The first question raised by the physician in the case presented is whether he should retain the patient in light of the anger aroused in him by the situation. The physician's anger stems from two sources: first, the mother's refusal to allow the child to be treated with antibiotics or to be immunized on religious grounds. The second source is the referral of the patient/family by a colleague who did not notify the physician of the possible visit thus leading the physician to feel "set up."

The anger directed toward the mother who will not allow antibiotic therapy for the child's otitis media can be readily understood, especially in light of the child's resultant hearing loss. The mother has not ruled out the therapy recommended by the physician, but she has stated that she must wait for direction from God as to whether or not to have the prescription filled. The mother, furthermore, has stated that she and her husband recently had a change in their religious beliefs and they no longer believe in immunization for their children. The situation which confronts the physician is how to provide adequate and appropriate medical care to the child while respecting the parents' religious beliefs.

The doctor cannot force the parents to have the children immunized since parents have the right to withhold immunizations from their children on religious grounds. Although schools prefer that children be protected from communicable diseases, children may be exempted from immunizations with a written statement from parents stating their religious objections (Ohio Department of Health, Bureau of Preventive Medicine, 1978). The physician might decide to pursue legal intervention if the antibiotics are not given to the child, but he must weigh the benefits and harms which could accrue from his actions. If he did pursue the legal avenue, he most likely would lose any possibility for follow-up with this family. Having retained the family as patients, he has kept the door open for future visits and additional opportunities for discussion with the family. At the same time he is able to keep tabs on the children's health. Since he does state in the incident that the otitis is resolving, he may choose to defer pressing the mother to administer antibiotic therapy on secular, scientific grounds until she perceives God's will.

In trying to resolve the problem, the physician listed five alternative courses of action. The path which he chose was a highly utilitarian one, and is really a sixth alternative since it differs from those listed. In his course of action, he maintained his professional and personal integrity by expressing his concerns to the mother while respecting her religious views, at least this time. While his informing her that he would continue to encourage her to have the children immunized in the future was admirably honest, there are two possible problems inherent in his "encouragement." The first is he may become overly vigorous, that is, coercive. Second, the mother may resent his "encouragement" and view it as a lack of respect for her beliefs and ultimately for her as a person. For the present time, however, he seems to have handled the situation appropriately.

The anger at the colleague stems from the physician's feeling "set up" in a situation that might be considered a breach of professional etiquette. It is difficult to assess the intentions of the colleague without talking with him directly, therefore a direct approach—which need not be equivalent to confrontation—seems reasonable. The referring physician may have thought the physician relating the incident had insights which would make him more understanding of the family and their needs. It would be appropriate to request notification of a referral—especially a difficult case—prior to the visit by the patient. The physician does not say whether he would have handled the situation differently if he had been notified of the visit beforehand or whether he simply resented the lack of courtesy and the feeling of being put on the spot.

The larger issue raised by this case is patient autonomy and its relationship to proxy consent for minors by parents juxtaposed with medical paternalism. In other words, should parents have the right to make decisions for their children which may, from the physician's perspective, jeopardize the child's future health? In this particular case, the decisions by the mother not to immunize the children and not to give antibiotic treatment for otitis media until she had discerned God's will were based on a relatively recent change in religious beliefs. It would be difficult for a physician under these circumstances not to take a paternalistic stance to protect the child's present and future health. Since the child at age three-and-one-half is not mature enough to decide for or against medical therapy, someone else clearly must make the decision. Consent is normally given in these instances by the parent, but the situation is greatly complicated if the physician disagrees with the parent's decision. In a similar circumstance involving Jehovah's Witnesses in which a child's life is threatened unless blood products are administered, the physician may appeal to the court to override the parents' wishes. In the past, courts have refused to permit Jehovah's Witnesses to decline blood transfusions for their children if the transfusions have been deemed medically necessary (Beauchamp & Childress, 1979; George, Edmark & Jones, 1976).

The physician is caught in the position of trying to juggle competing claims, namely respecting the family's autonomy and maintaining his own integrity in caring for the child to the best of his ability. The situation is rife with the potential for coercion and alienation: if the physician gives in to the temptation to coerce the parent to accept his views regarding medical care (paternalism), he may alienate her, thus the child will be lost to follow-up. Similarly, if the principle of autonomy is important to the physician, he will have violated his own principle by applying pressure to the parent. The circumstances surrounding the case, namely the differences in religious beliefs and attitudes toward medial therapies of the parents and the physician, require that the doctor think through the possibilities for future interaction and potential conflict with the parents. He needs to be aware of how far he is willing to compromise regarding medical treatment of the children. He may want to seek legal counsel to be prepared to deal with a more critical situation should it arise.

For the present, it can be said that the physician in this particular case handled a difficult situation well, especially since he has kept open opportunities for future contact.

Joy D. Skeel, B. S. Nsg., M. Div.
Instructor in Medical Humanities, Department of Psychiatry
Instructor in Medicine, Department of Medicine
Medical College of Ohio at Toledo
Toledo, Ohio

References

Beauchamp, T. L., & Childress, J. F. Principles of biomedical ethics. New York: Oxford University Press, 1979.

George, T., Edmark, R., & Jones, T. Issues involved with surgery on Jehovah's Witnesses. In S. Gorovitz, A. Jameston, R. Macklin, J. O'Conner, E. Perrin, B. St. Clair, & S. Sherwin (Eds.), *Moral problems in medicine*. Englewood Cliffs, N.J.: Prentice-Hall, 1976.

Ohio Department of Health, Bureau of Preventive Medicine. *Immunization Recommendations and Requirements*, 1978.

Suggested Reading

Devorkin, G. Paternalism. In S. Gorovitz, A. Jameston, R. Macklin, J. O'Conner, E. Perrin, B. St. Clair, & S. Sherwin (Eds.), *Moral problems in medicine*. Englewood Cliffs, N.J.: Prentice-Hall, 1976.

Commentary

Four important questions emerge from this case: the ethical responsibility of this physician toward the family unit; the ethical responsibility of the referring physician toward his colleague; the ethical responsibility of the parents toward the children; and the emotional atmosphere that was created as a result of this incident.

I would hold that this physician's response was within the range of ethical behavior toward his patient. Any satisfactory account of the doctor–patient relationship would hold that the physician may refuse to offer a particular treatment, or may refuse to treat a particular patient, if doing so would involve him in a violation of his own moral values; for example, as would occur with a Roman Catholic physician asked to perform an abortion. However, from the physician's point of view, would failure to immunize the child, in fact, be *immoral?* It would certainly be imprudent to a high degree; but it would be hard to specify a particular moral principle or moral value which this behavior would violate. (Medical science in and of itself should probably not be construed as a moral standard of behavior.) Therefore, this physician made his own value stance clear but did not reject the family outright.

The physician's responsibility is colored by the issue of whether these parents have satisfactorily discharged their own moral obligations to the children. In the most extreme situation, where actual child abuse or neglect is present, the physician would be obligated both morally and legally to report the family to child protection authorities. To the medical mind, failure to immunize seems to constitute blatant child neglect; but the rest of society may not share this view. In Virginia, for example, the child abuse and neglect statute specifically excludes jurisdiction when medical care is withheld for bona fide religious beliefs.

By agreeing, on his own terms, to continue treating this family, the physician committed no immoral action and left the gate open for future renegotiation of the doctor–patient relationship. This family has converted its religious beliefs once; they may again. Or it may be possible to present the recommendations for treatment in terms that do not conflict with the religious beliefs (for example, if immunizations are seen as assisting the body's own natural health-maintaining mechanisms). But these renegotiations will occur only in an established atmosphere of trust and acceptance. Refusing to care for the family unless they did it "his way," or trying heavy-handedly to challenge the validity of their religious views, would have made this impossible.

What, then, was the responsibility of the colleague who initiated the referral? Very little imagination would seem to be required to picture how this physician would feel when the mother disclosed her attitudes. At best, the colleague ought not to have referred the family at all without the expressed consent of the physician; at worst, he should have at least warned the physician of this family's views before they arrived in his office. Simple golden-rule ethics demand no less.

The colleague's responsibility becomes particularly important in light of the emotional atmosphere that was created by the interview. Anger was the most prominent emotion experienced by the physician, and this occurred despite the fact that the mother, according to the account, expressed herself in a generally pleasant manner. The anger, therefore, was primarily aroused by the absent colleague and by the feeling of having been "set up." I suspect that it was primarily this anger, rather than a particular devotion to either "medical science" or to his own religious values, that almost led the physician to consider rejecting the family, preaching to them patronizingly, or washing his hands of responsibility. Fortunately, and no thanks to the colleague, he managed to avoid these temptations. Seeing clearly from the first that the anger was directed at the colleague and not at the mother might have made his choice easier.

Howard Brody, M.D., Ph.D
Assistant Professor, Family Practice and Philosophy
Assistant Coordinator, Medical Humanities Program
Michigan State University
East Lansing, Michigan

Suggested Readings

Blustein, J. On children and proxy consent. *Journal of Medical Ethics,* 1978, 4, 138–140.
Shaw, A. Dilemmas of "informed consent" in children. *New England Journal of Medicine,* 1973, 289, 885–890.

IV / The Practice

The practice of family medicine involves more than the application of medical knowledge. As we have seen in the previous three sections, it also involves certain issues in the training of family physicians as well as issues engendered in the relationships with other physicians, nonphysician professionals, and patients. In addition, the practicing family physician must enter other worlds that the uninitiated may not expect, such as business, law, and ethics. Having sufficient knowledge and expertise to appropriately function in these areas is essential to the success of any family practice. The necessity of entering these diverse arenas adds further complexity to the role of the family physician and may result in many critical incidents. In recognition of their complexity and importance, most family practice residency programs include training in practice management, ethics, and medicolegal issues.

The incidents which have been placed under the rubric of "The Practice" reflect issues arising not only out of the family physician's traditional role but from these other areas as well. To the reader it may seem that some of these incidents should have been placed in other sections. While the issues clearly do overlap, these incidents justified a separate section because they arise as a result of what the physician does or does not do in the course of his practice. Clear resolution of the issues evolving from these incidents is of key importance because how the physician resolves these incidents intrapersonally determines how he will practice in the future.

These incidents arise out of situations which demand quick responses and are difficult to anticipate. In perusing this section, the reader should ask himself not only whether the incidents were handled properly but whether there are alternate solutions. Could similar situations and their solutions be anticipated, or, better, prevented in his own practice? Many of these incidents point up the importance of communicating to others the physician's personal and professional policies and standards. The reader might ask himself if he is accomplishing this communication with others. These incidents also invariably produced emotional strain and conflict between and within each of the parties involved. It may be helpful for the reader to analyze how the authors and commentators handle these emotionally painful situations and, thus, begin to consider his own style of coping.

The incidents and commentaries in this section should be particularly helpful to new practitioners and advanced trainees in the health profession, for they are in a position of setting up a practice and thus instituting new policies and procedures of their own. For the more experienced practitioners, consideration of these issues can be valuable to the ongoing evaluation of their practice experiences.

The Editors

27 / All in the Family
Confidentiality and Family Members

Background

A 67-year-old retired spinster schoolteacher was hospitalized for radiotherapy to palliate metastatic breast disease. The patient was beloved by the entire small community where she had resided and taught school for nearly half a century. Through the years, she had received numerous awards for community service and dedication to her profession. She was a charming and witty individual who was well aware of her diagnosis and was managing it beautifully by utilizing subtle denial mechanisms. My rapport with the patient was excellent. Her response to treatment was actually quite dramatic, and after a period of two weeks, she was ready for dismissal.

The Incident

On the afternoon prior to the patient's planned hospital discharge, an unscheduled visitor came to my office insisting she needed to speak to me about a highly personal matter. The visitor was an elderly lady who informed me that she was the older sister and only living relative of my hospitalized cancer patient. I was somewhat shocked since I had been led to believe that my patient had no surviving blood relatives. She had, in fact, adopted the entire community as her family. The visitor seemed sincere and asked that I provide details of her sister's condition in order that she might be better prepared to aid her with both her physical illness and her personal affairs. I complied with her request, actually feeling relieved that there was someone to share this burden with me.

The following morning I visited my patient in the hospital and found her profoundly irate for the first time ever. She informed me that she had not been on speaking terms with her sister for many years, that she considered her sister to be a cunning and untrustworthy individual, and that she thoroughly resented her sister having knowledge of her personal affairs and illness. Apparently the older sister had gone directly from my office to the hospital, gloated, and informed the patient that I had shared all this information with her.

From that day forward, the patient's personality was the exact opposite of the one I had known for many years. She remained depressed, agitated, uncooperative, and at times combative. She refused to leave the hospital or make any effort to resume a meaningful existence. Her condition rapidly deteriorated, and she expired approximately four weeks following the critical incident.

Discussion

This vignette directs our attention to several key issues. How might I have avoided the conflict by better protecting the confidentiality of my relationship with the patient? Is a physician ever really justified in violating the principle of confidentiality? How does the "need to know" policy, employed by the military and government in protecting confidential information, apply to the physician? In terms of confidentiality, how does practice in a small community differ from practice in a metropolitan area? What similarities exist? In this situation, should I have withdrawn in hope that another physician might better have brought comfort to the patient in her final days?

The above story occurred during the early days of my medical practice. Despite the agony and pain it inflicted, it remains one of the great teaching and learning experiences I have encountered. Time has done little to dull the impact.

Commentary

The ethical questions raised by this case are reasonably clear. Confidentiality is a duty owed to the patient by the doctor as part of the physician–patient relationship. Confidentiality may be justified for the following reasons: (1) the right to privacy of the patient; (2) the implied promise of confidentiality based on past cultural practices in medicine which the patient has the right to assume upon entering the relationship; and (3) for utilitarian reasons, namely, that in the absence of confidentiality, patients would be unwilling to reveal many sensitive matters to their physicians and the decreased quality of care resulting would lead to an increase of human misery.

Virtually all commentators regard confidentiality as a qualified rather than as an absolute duty. Beauchamp and Childress (1979) characterize it as a *prima facie* duty, a duty which is generally binding but which may, in special circumstances, be overridden by a competing, stronger duty. The burden of proof, then, is upon the individual who would violate a *prima facie* duty; he is obligated to show, first, that some other conflicting duty exists, and second, that the other duty should be regarded as the stronger one.

Averting a clear danger to the public welfare and protecting the life or safety of another individual is the clearest example of a duty that overrides the patient's right to confidentiality. Thus, reporting communicable disease cases even over the objections of the patient or notifying the police of a homicide threat reported by a patient in confidence are ethically justifiable examples of overriding confidentiality. More difficult cases arise when the harm to be prevented is less severe, or when there is less likelihood that maintaining confidentiality will actually result in harm.

None of these valid reasons for overriding confidentiality is present in the case of the schoolteacher. The physician might have reasoned that, since in the vast majority of cases patients voluntarily permit the physician to disclose medical information to members of their immediate families, this patient would give similar consent for her sister. In this assumption he was, of course, mistaken, and since nothing would have been lost by delaying his answer to the sister's questions until he had checked with the patient herself, proceeding to act on this unproven assumption was not appropriate. Alternatively, the physician might have reasoned that this sister could offer needed support and comfort in this instance of terminal disease, and thus the benefit to the patient outweighed the duty to maintain confidentiality. Not only was this prediction unsound, but the purported benefit was insufficient to justify the violation of a *prima facie* duty. The patient herself was the one to judge whether she valued her privacy more or less than any assistance she might get from the sister. Finally, the physician may have based his actions upon a presumed "need to know" on the part of the family of a terminally ill person. (This sense of a duty to inform the family may have arisen historically from the practice of concealing terminal diagnoses from patients but disclosing the truth to the family instead; fortunately, this practice of withholding information from the patient is declining.) But this supposed "need" is secondary to the rights of the patient within the doctor–patient relationship. In case of a conflict between family and patient interests, where the behavioral insights and the interpersonal skills of the physician cannot resolve the conflict in a mutually acceptable fashion, the physician must go along with his overriding duty to the patient.

Medical practice in a small town increases the vigilence that a physician must exercise in order to maintain confidentiality, but does not change the strength of the obligation to maintain confidentiality.

We must conclude, then, that the physician in this case, however well-intentioned, committed a serious ethical error. What should he have done next? One wishes the case description provided more detail on precisely how he approached the patient afterwards. Did he openly acknowledge his error, emphasize his good intentions, and offer apology? Or did he try to go on as if nothing had happened? Had he adopted the former course, it seems highly unlikely that a relationship based on past trust and mutual respect would be irrevocably shattered merely as the result of this one honest mistake. Alternatively, the severity of this patient's reaction may have been rooted deep in the history of this traumatic relationship with the sister. Perhaps the patient would have fallen into an identical depression from the sister's visit alone, even had the physician maintained confidentiality.

This case illustrates the dangers of uncritically applying concepts and behavior that are appropriate to "normal" families to idiosyncratic or unusual situations. (Ironically, in this case the good family physician can be too "family-oriented" and thus neglect his ethical duty to the patient as an individual.) Imagine what would have happened had this patient lapsed into a coma and had this sister appeared as the physician was trying to decide on further treatment. Legally, the sister is the next of kin and is the appropriate party to give or withhold consent for treatment on the patient's behalf, but ethically, any of a number of the patient's friends in the town could better have represented her true viewpoint and interests. We can see the value of "living will" proposals such as those of Bok (1976) and Relman (1979), which would allow the patient to designate an agent of his or her choosing to make terminal care decisions, should the patient later become incompetent to do so.

An intriguing feature of this case is the way that, despite the physician's good intentions, an action which turned out to be a violation of an ethical duty also had a negative impact therapeutically on the patient's physical condition. It is widely reported in the psychosomatic literature that exacerbations of chronic diseases, such as cancer, can be caused by depression or hopelessness. Winslade (1978) notes in his analysis of confidentiality that the ability to control aspects of one's life, specifically the sort of information about oneself that others are given, is a crucial feature of the right of privacy on which confidentiality is based. Cassell (1976), in his thoughtful work on the physician–patient relationship in chronic disease, emphasizes the concept of mastery and control over the symptoms of illness and over the impact that illness has on one's life, even when no cure is possible. Cassell argues that treatment strategies that decrease the patient's own sense of mastery and control lead to worsening of the course of illness. Brody and Waters (1980) contend that these changes are direct changes, analogous to the placebo effect, produced by the altered meaning that the illness experience assumes for the patient. These hypotheses, applied to the case of the schoolteacher, would have led to the prediction that this violation of confidentiality would produce a sharply decreased sense of control over herself and her situation and that this, in turn, would produce an exacerbation of symptoms and diminished resistance to the effects of the cancer. While much more dramatic in this case than usual, this reminder of the connection between attitudes and physical states points out that ethics and clinical medicine do not occupy separate, watertight compartments. Ethics, at its base, has to do with respect for the individual autonomy and dignity of persons, and this respect, or its absence, can also have direct clinical and therapeutic implications.

In preparing this commentary I was assisted by a group discussion of the incident among the faculty of the Department of Family Practice, Michigan State University, and was especially aided by comments from Anne Cunningham, Linda Garcia-Shelton, Roy Gerard, and James Hudson.

Howard Brody, M.D., Ph.D.
Assistant Professor, Family Practice and Philosophy
Assistant Coordinator, Medical Humanities Program
Michigan State University
East Lansing, Michigan

References
Beauchamp, T. L., & Childress, J. F. *Principles of biomedical ethics*. New York: Oxford University Press, 1979.
Bok, S. Personal directions for care at the end of life. *New England Journal of Medicine*, 1976, *295*, 367–369.
Brody, H., & Waters, D. B. Diagnosis is treatment. *Journal of Family Practice*, 1980, *10*, 445–449.
Cassell, E. J. *The healer's art: A new approach to the doctor–patient relationship*. Philadelphia: Lippincott, 1976.
Relman, A. S. Michigan's sensible "living will." *New England Journal of Medicine*, 1979, *300*, 1270–1271.
Winslade, W. J. Confidentiality. In W. T. Reich (Ed.), *Encyclopedia of bioethics* (Vol. 1). New York: Free Press, 1978.

Commentary

My comments about the issues relating to this 67-year-old lady with breast cancer will fall into two general categories: the first group will address the questions raised by the writer of the critical incident; the second group of comments are issues that touch on my sensitivity.

The author's first question is, "How might I have avoided the conflict by better protecting the confidentiality of my relationship with the patient?" In retrospect, the conflict could have been avoided by checking with the patient before talking about her medical condition with anyone. This would have allowed her to be in control of the release of information.

"Is the physician ever really justified in violating the principle of confidentiality?" At times one is tempted to violate the principles of confidentiality, as in the following examples:

1. The 16-year-old driver that you treat in the emergency room at 2 A.M. who is drunk, involved in an accident, and doesn't want his parents called.
2. The person who is mentally ill and is potentially dangerous.

While I was in the Navy, a Marine told me that he was going to kill his lieutenant. I told him that I would tell his lieutenant and then did, which was an open violation of his confidentiality.

The underlying principle of violation of confidentiality is that there is apparent overwhelming evidence that the patient or someone else will be harmed if precautions are not taken. Another category for information release without the authority of the patient would be when the patient is not able to make a rational decision for himself, such as being in a state of emotional or physical shock or unconsciousness. Fortunately, when the physician feels the need to release information and shares these feelings with the patient, the outcome is usually with the consent of the patient. For example, I had one patient who did not want his wife to know he had metastatic prostate cancer. After about a year, when the disease was causing serious symptoms, I felt he needed to share the information with his wife. I asked him to reconsider and told him that if he did not choose to share the information, he should see another doctor and I would tell his wife over his objections. He reconsidered and discussed his illness with her.

"In terms of confidentiality, how does practice in a small community differ from practice in a metropolitan area?" Having practiced medicine in both a small community and in a metropolitan area, I feel the principles of confidentiality are the same. In a small community, one is more likely to know and encounter the significant family members and friends of the patient. If confidentiality is breached inappropriately in a small town, one is more likely to lose credibility with many people because of the more total sharing of information in smaller groups.

As with most critical incidents with patients, rights and wrongs are generally not zero or 100 percent. Given the situation described and given the question, "Should I have withdrawn in hopes another physician might better have brought comfort to the patient in her final days?", I feel the best solution to pursue initially would have been to talk directly and openly with her when both the physician and patient appeared to be able to talk, think, and interact openly, candidly, and nonjudgmentally. I believe that *critical decisions of patients should generally be made with the patient (who is capable and informed) and not for them*. Translating this philosophy into action, I would say to the patient, "I was wrong to tell your sister. Would you forgive me? Do you want me to continue to be your doctor? Should I arrange for another doctor to care for you because of my mistake?" If the patient chose another doctor, I would arrange for the transfer. If she continued to have me as her physician, I would do my best to take care of her and her illness. It would also be necessary to establish rules of communication acceptable to both of us.

The second set of comments are issues that I feel are within the critical incident that weren't explicitly raised by the author, who I feel demonstrates strength in sharing the critical incident. When one finds oneself in a difficult situation which arouses strong feelings, a discussion with peers is often helpful for ventilation and, perhaps more important, for problem-solving. In addition, at times spouses are excellent resources for moral-ethical decisions.

The following thoughts of other people are also pertinent:

Norman Cousins is one of our modern moral philosophers. In his battle with ankylosing spondylitis, he felt that "the principle contribution made by my doctor to the taming, and possibly the conquest, of my illness was that he encouraged me to believe I was a respected partner with him in the total undertaking" (Cousins, 1976, p. 1463).

The AMA Principles of Medical Ethics (1980) approved by the House of Delegates, states: "A physician shall respect the rights of patients, of colleagues, and of other health professionals, and shall safeguard patient confidences within the constrains of law."

Each state has the opportunity, through its legislature, to issue guidelines about patient confidentiality. Most interpersonal patient confidentiality guidelines are, in fact, based on common law. In Ohio, for example, no explicit statute applies to sibling confidentiality (Ohio State Medical Association, undated).

The American College of Legal Medicine has not made a policy statement as yet about confidentiality. Personal correspondence with them reveals that they have not yet addressed this issue.

> The College has, in the past several years, addressed several issues of broad national concern in the legal aspects of medical practice and has even taken a position on a few of them. I must say, however, patient confidentiality has not been one of the subjects on which either the Board of Governors or the membership has felt required a position by the College [Reed, 1981].

My working guidelines of confidentiality are that a patient who is able to make informed decisions about himself has the right to determine to whom I may release information. Therefore, I discuss the issue with the patient and let him decide. If a 14-year-old fits these guidelines, then I would not discuss, fully and openly, his problems with anyone he does not direct or allow me to talk with, unless extenuating circumstances were involved, such as doing harm to himself or others.

Each physician develops his own ethic. Given the apparent paucity of legal direction in court cases and state statutes, you may want to check with appropriate legal counsel for your state requirements and, more important, his interpretations and guidance about any particularly tough situation.

Larry W. Johnson, M.D.
Associate Professor, Department of Family Medicine
Medical College of Ohio at Toledo
Toledo, Ohio

References

American Medical Association. *Principles of medical ethics*. Chicago: Author, 1980.

Cousins, N. Anatomy of an illness (as perceived by the patient). *New England Journal of Medicine*, December 23, 1976, *295*(26), 1458–1463.

Ohio State Medical Association. *Physician's guide to Ohio law*. Columbus, Ohio: Author. (Undated pamphlet.)

Reed, E. A. Personal correspondence. American College of Legal Medicine, January 27, 1981.

28 / Intrusion?

Patient Compliance, Unannounced House Calls, and Patient Anger

Background

The patient was a 28-year-old white single female with one child and had had an abortion two weeks before. The pathology report was "suggestive of trophoblastic disease" (i.e., hydatidiform mole). A beta subunit HCG was obtained which was high and consistent with a recent abortion. The patient and I agreed to follow the gynecologist's recommendation to check the beta subunit HCG every two weeks for a total of eight weeks. However, the patient did not come in until the eighth week, after I sent her a letter urging her to do so. She claimed she did not have a phone.

The Incident

The lab ran the beta subunit HCG but had technical problems and asked for another sample of blood. Rather than send a letter, which during the holiday season would take too much time, I made a home visit without notifying the patient. The patient was upset that I "treaded on her privacy." This made me feel angry because I did it for her well-being. She was angry and refused to come to the office. She did not accept my explanations of no phone by which to contact her and the urgency of getting the blood test. The final outcome was that there was a little serum left which the lab tested and found to be normal.

When the patient was told the result, she asked, "What was everyone so excited about?" The gynecologist suggested one more test, one month later, which the patient again refused.

Discussion

It is easy for a physician to become angry when a patient refuses to comply with what one is trying to do to help her. Yet stepping on her territory without permission elicited anger. Although I felt this was a risk, my anticipation was wrong, making a difficult situation even worse. Fortunately, there appears to be no disease. However, her health care may be jeopardized, at least with our clinic (she claims to be seeing another M.D./gynecologist). I wonder if this could have been avoided. Probably not, as there is more to this case than is able to be described here.

Commentary

The basic question the physician is asking in this incident is, "Why was the patient angry with me when I was just interested in assuring her well-being?" The physician's reaction to the patient's anger was anger directed at her for not understanding that his concern for her health was the motivating factor in his behavior. A communication problem exists. An evaluation of the physician–patient contract(s) and problem solving of the incidents arising in this scenario will permit us to see what went wrong.

It is unclear from the information provided whether this physician and patient had established a relationship and contract prior to the termination of the pregnancy. For purposes of discussion, we will assume the first contact between the two individuals was at the time of the termination of the pregnancy. At that time, some discussion or information sheet regarding the nature of the services to be provided by the physician and his office staff to this patient and the patient's obligation to the physician should have transpired; thus, an initial contract is formulated.

Plans for completing this patient's data base should have been determined at that time. Dr. Medalie (1978) has devoted a chapter to a complete data base from which individuals can extract components appropriate for their practice. While collecting this data base, current and potential psychosocial problems are identified which may have prevented the communication problems that occurred in this scenario. Ernest Yuh-Ting Yen (1980) stresses the importance of assessing the nonmedical aspects of the individual and family settings. In this instance, the impact of termination of the pregnancy on this individual and her family must be assessed.

Upon receipt of the pathology report, a second problem arises (possible hydatidiform mole) requiring a modification of the original treatment plan and contract to the extent of frequent lab work and more contact with the physician. At this time, an assessment of the patient's ability to meet the time and financial obligations necessitated by this change is required. This assessment could be done via telephone or in the office with the physician or his nurse (the latter is preferable). It is imperative that the patient understand the importance of the therapy plan and the seriousness of the possible disease and be allowed to express any concerns about the impact of this plan on her current life situation. For example, she may be trying to forget the pregnancy and may not be equipped to handle the constant reminders of it generated by visiting the lab and the physician's office. This conflict may have to be dealt with before any tests are done, or may be addressed concurrently with the revised medical treatment plan. Then, the therapy plan can be modified to meet both the physician's goals and the patient's expectations; a second (modified) contract is formulated.

From the description of the planned therapy, we can assume that the diagnosis of hydatidiform mole is probably not highly suspected. If it were, a different plan would probably have been recommended, for example, initial chest x-ray followed by biweekly quantitative beta subunit HCG's until negative, and then monthly until a year from the initial evaluation, as recommended by Danforth (1977).

We now return to the scenario with the patient agreeing to the second or modified contract. With this established, the physician's office would know if the patient did not present for laboratory work before the eight weeks had elapsed. Problems with maintaining the biweekly visits could be addressed and appropriately resolved by telephone, letter, or office visits.

The next problem that surfaced is what to do when a laboratory test needs to be repeated. This is a fairly common problem that usually creates little more than some minor inconveniences in individual schedules. The patient's anger at being informed of this was probably more directed at the way in which she was informed—by an unannounced home visit. Usually, a simple explanation of the problem (tube broke, machine error, etc.) will suffice to encourage the patient to repeat the test at no additional charge. However, before the repeat is requested the lab should be sure it cannot perform the test on any specimen it may have left. Whether the laboratory or the physician is responsible for notifying the patient is an interesting question that we do not have the time to address here.

The unannounced home visit would not be necessary if the above listed process had occurred. Most patients do not expect a house call unless such a provision is in the original contract or they specifically ask for one. Her offense and anger at such a visit is certainly understandable as a violation of her privacy. Her anger at the process (home visit) then escalated to the content (repeat lab test) and she refused to come in. If this visit was deemed necessary by the physician, some introductory, nonthreatening remarks regarding the importance of the visit should have been made when the patient answered the door. Then the patient would most likely have accepted the visit and its projected outcome of repeat lab test. Her apparent lack of concern expressed when told the repeat lab test was negative was merely a reinforcement of her anger about the home visit and strengthened her position ("I told you that test wasn't necessary"). Her apparent lack of concern could also be related to her not understanding the suspected disease and the need for evaluation, or could be an expression of her denying having the disease. These possibilities imply the need for more information to be gathered in these areas and appropriate patient education provided. While a patient has the right to refuse treatment or procedures, Medalie (1978) states that most experienced physicians use the best "medicine" in their practice ("the doctor") to encourage compliance. Obviously, this centers around having a "good" doctor–patient relationship, which is not present here.

While we see how this situation may have been prevented by fostering a therapeutic doctor–patient relationship, obtaining a complete data base, and establishing contracts, we are left with the present situation. Where do we go from here with the patient angry at her doctor, seemingly unconcerned about the potential seriousness of her medical problem, and a physician angry at the patient for not understanding his intentions? The critical question is, "What does the physician want to do with this situation?" If he feels unable to continue to provide care for this patient, another physician should be found; if the patient is not interested in continuing with this physician, another should be found. If he wants to continue to provide care for this patient and she concurs, they need to reestablish a more appropriate doctor–patient relationship, and arrangements should be made for this. An appointment with the inclusion of a process observer such as another physician or office nurse to facilitate open communication and contract agreement is the first step.

If the physician is in training, he should *not* be allowed to merely transfer the patient's care. His program needs to provide the necessary educational resources and support for him and the patient to facilitate reestablishing a more appropriate doctor–patient relationship. Specifically, the resident must become more cognizant of the aspects of a "good" doctor–patient relationship and be attentive to these factors when dealing with his patients. To let this initial aspect of a physician's development be discarded by transferring doctors is inappropriate in any residency program. Additional counseling or therapy that is needed for either resident or patient can be provided either within or outside the program, but a mechanism for such should be established.

This clinical scenario, like similar ones, really demonstrates many aspects of the art of medicine. We often forget about good communication skills, listening skills, and empathy that we were exposed to as medical students. Establishing an appropriate doctor–patient relationship that both parties can live with is the cornerstone of health care delivery no matter what discipline of medicine one practices. Attention to the "human aspects" can often do more than the best science in medicine to promote health.

Chris D. Marquart, M.D.
Professor and Chairman, Council of Family Medicine
Northeastern Ohio Universities College of Medicine
Rootstown, Ohio

References
Danforth, D. N. *Obstetrics and gynecology* (3rd ed.). New York: Harper and Row, 1977.
Medalie, J. E. *Family medicine, principles and applications*. Baltimore: Williams & Wilkins, 1978.
Yuh-Ting Yen, E. *Review and assessment in family practice*. New York: Appleton-Century-Crofts, 1980.

Suggested Readings
Ingelfinger, E. J. Arrogance. *New England Journal of Medicine*, June 28, 1979, *303*(26), 1507–1510.
Milion, T. *Medical behavioral science*. Philadelphia: Saunders, 1975.

Commentary

This critical incident raises a number of issues important to the doctor–patient relationship and the provision of good health care, namely, the contract between the physician and the patient, compliance with medical regimen, the use of the house call, emotional responses on both parts when there is a misunderstanding, and the necessity of understanding the psychosocial aspects of the patient's life. Let us look at each of these issues in light of this incident and the questions raised by the physician.

It is unclear whether the physician had been taking care of the patient for a period of time or whether he had assumed her care subsequent to the abortion. For the sake of discussion, I will assume the latter. At this time the physician is faced with a patient who had a recent abortion and now has a pathology report suggestive of a serious disease. With this in mind, the physician needs to establish rapport with the patient and also develop a contract with her to take care of this problem. Szasz and Hollender (1956) described the model of mutual participation which requires that "the participants (1) have approximately equal power, (2) be mutually interdependent (i.e., need each other), and (3) engage in activity that will be mutually satisfying to both" (p. 587).

It seems to me that this physician is willing to share the power with the patient, as he states that they mutually agreed to follow the gynecologist's recommendation. However, when one party does not assume their share of the power, as in the case of this patient, the physician may then have needed to assert the power of his expertise and take more immediate action to discuss this with her. It is important that the physician understand why the patient did not assume her share of the responsibility for her health care, as this will influence how the physician will need to handle the patient's care.

Mutual interdependence may be more apparent to the physician, who needs patients in order to exercise his skill and knowledge, than it may be to the patient. It may be difficult for her to accept that she may have a serious disease, or she may no longer feel she needs the physician if obtaining an abortion was viewed as the resolution of her problem. It seems to me that establishing a mutual interdependence in this case can occur only with an understanding of the patient's feelings and current situation as well as carefully explaining the physician's concerns about her health. Unless she is aware and accepts that she needs the physician's help, she will be unable to allow this interdependence to occur.

The third criterion of engaging in activity that will be mutually satisfying may have some difficulties in this case. If this woman finds out she has a serious illness, it may not be "satisfying" to her, and this is what faces her at the initiation of the contract. The physician needs to approach this from the standpoint of working together on the mutual goal of maintaining her health, which will promise long-range satisfaction for her. And part of this is the early detection of disease in order to provide effective treatment.

There are also certain practical issues which need to be dealt with at the time of negotiating a contract, such as expectations concerning appointments, payment of fees, and mutual expectations regarding how services will be provided. In addition to gathering medical history, it is also appropriate to begin asking questions about the patient's life situation. If it becomes known at this time that the patient does not have a telephone, as in this case, the physician or another member of the health care team can request a number where a message can be left in the event that the physician's office needs to reach her. Occasionally, it may be necessary to cancel or change the patient's appointment time. If the patient has no alternative number, this presents an opportunity to problem-solve with the patient around this issue, as it is at times essential that the physician be able to reach a patient promptly. Had this been done, the unannounced house call may not have occurred or may have been accepted more positively by the patient.

Let us turn to the issue of compliance. Stone (1979) found that patients must know what recommendations have been made in order to comply. He stated that the aspects of the physician–patient interaction which affect compliance are (1) the effectiveness with which the information is given and (2) the interpersonal message sent by the physician to the patient. It is difficult to evaluate the interaction between the physician and the patient in this incident, except that the patient did not seem to understand or accept the seriousness of the condition, as demonstrated by her reaction when the test was found to be normal, stating, "What was everyone so excited about?" In any case of noncompliance, it seems to me that both the physician and the patient need to look at the interaction to determine where the breakdown in communication occurred. I would suggest, through my own clinical experience, that most difficulties in communication occur because of the interpersonal message conveyed rather than the effectiveness of the presentation. Generally, when strong feelings are evoked in a patient, it is then difficult for him or her to hear a rational message. This is the art of medicine: to be aware of the verbal and nonverbal messages that the patient conveys, to be aware of one's own feelings and reactions, and to use this information in the best interests of the patient (Engel, 1977). This may improve communication, compliance, and satisfaction.

In this case the physician was also guilty of not complying with the contract. To establish a contract that a certain test will be done every two weeks for a total of eight weeks and then to allow most of this time to elapse before sending a letter to the patient is certainly not appropriate follow-up nor does it give reinforcement of the physician's concern. It is certainly difficult for a busy physician to be aware of every patient who does not appear for lab work. This may have to be followed by another member of the health care team who can alert the physician immediately when a patient does not attend so that contact can be made promptly. This response by a physician demonstrates his concern and also says to the patient, "Our contract is important to me and so are you." We must note that when the patient was contacted to return for tests, she did respond.

Considering the issues previously discussed, my feeling is that the unannounced house call was inappropriate and was probably related to the physician's feelings of guilt. In our society unannounced visits from authority figures are usually negative, as in the case of protective service workers, bill collectors, process servers, or the police. I am not surprised that the patient was upset and felt that her privacy had been invaded. The patient may also have felt confused since the doctor did not notify her or make a house call during the eight weeks when she did not appear for the test. His appearance at her door after the test may have been frightening, and many people react to fear with anger.

Family medicine, as delineated by McWhinney(1981), advocates the use of the house call in several situations: the assessment and/or management of acute illness; the management of patients discharged from the hospital; the management of patients with chronic diseases; the management of patients with terminal illness; and the assessment of home conditions and family functions. Home visits are made upon the request of the patient when the doctor deems them appropriate or when they are planned and scheduled with the family to assure their privacy. In this case the house call was neither planned nor requested. It may have been more appropriate for the physician to send one of his nurses, office personnel, or even a public health nurse. If this was not feasible, a telegram may have been sent requesting that the patient contact the physician. Any of these means of conveying a message may have been less threatening to the patient. It is my impression that the writer of the incident was either a resident or a newly practicing physician who may have been idealistic as well as frightened that he could be blamed for a bad outcome in this case.

The issue of the emotional responses of both parties when there is a misunderstanding is relevant to the outcome of this incident. While we do not know specifically why the patient did not comply, I would assume that in part she was defensively using denial, either associated with the abortion and/or the possibility of a serious illness. We have no information regarding her psychological state, current life stresses, or characteristic patterns of reaction. Her anger at the doctor's house call was probably justified from her perspective. The physician, it seems, may have felt guilty and concerned at his lack of follow-up and may not have been aware of his feelings. When the patient responded angrily, the physician also felt angry because he had made the visit for the patient's well-being. While this is true on one level, on a deeper level the visit was made to assuage his feelings of guilt and fear. At this point we have two angry people, which makes problem-solving very difficult. Had the physician been aware of his own feelings of guilt, he might have been able to control his anger and respond to what the patient was feeling, namely intruded upon and perhaps frightened. It may have been necessary to allow her to ventilate her feelings and then apologize to her for the intrustion. He could explain that he was concerned about having an accurate test as soon as possible. The physician might then, or at some later time, depending on the reactions of the patient, discuss this situation and determine whether they could resume a satisfactory working relationship. The physician and patient might need to renegotiate their original contract, as they have gathered new information about each other and about potential problem situations. In this incident the patient chose to seek her medical care elsewhere, which was of concern to the physician. He wonders if this could have been avoided and says, "Probably not, as there is more to this case than is able to be described here." Without this information it is difficult to consider whether this outcome could have been avoided, but I would like to think it could have been prevented with some initial understanding between the patient and the physician around the issues already discussed.

The last point I would like to make involves the importance of the physician having an understanding of the psychosocial aspects of the patient's life.

Ireton and Cassata (1976, p. 155) state that "an essential attitude is the physician's willingness to view the patient presenting symptoms and signs as possible indicators of emotional stress as well as of organic disease at the outset." In order to develop this attitude, it is essential that the physician have a means of collecting and organizing all the data that will provide an understanding of the patient's total life situation. Ireton and Cassata propose a Psychological Systems Review as a means of integrating all the information about the patient including emotional status, life situation, and personality style. They stress that the physician needs to understand the current functioning as well as the patient's overall personality, major life stresses, and adaptive operations in order to effectively take care of the patient. I feel that the physician in the incident would have had less difficulty with this patient if he had developed such a review. He would then have been able to anticipate more accurately the reactions of the patient and could have predicated his actions on a clearer understanding of the needs of the patient.

The emphasis and training in family medicine affords many opportunities to learn the techniques and develop the skills to do this kind of assessment and use it effectively in patient care. Behavioral science training is available in most residency programs, but in order to be effective, the behavioral science curriculum needs to be integrated into the total curriculum and receive the support of medical faculty. While providing good medical care is essential, it is also essential for a physician to understand himself and his patients as people.

Rita L. Hermann, M.S.S.W.
Assistant Professor
Department of Family Medicine
Medical College of Ohio at Toledo
Toledo, Ohio

References

Engel, G. L. The care of the patient: Art or science? *The Johns Hopkins Medical Journal*, 1977, *140*, 222–232.

Ireton, H. R., & Cassata, D. M. A psychological systems review. *The Journal of Family Practice*, 1976, *3*, 155–159.

McWhinney, I. R. *An introduction to family medicine*. New York: Oxford University Press, 1981.

Stone, F. C. Patient compliance and the role of the expert. *Journal of Social Issues*, 1979, *35*, 34–59.

Szasz, T. S., & Hollender, M. H. A contribution to the philosophy of medicine: The basic models of the doctor–patient relationship. *Archives of Internal Medicine*, 1956, *97*, 585–592.

29 / My Partner's Keeper
Interphysician Communication and Patient Care

Background

I was scheduled for a follow-up appointment to reassess oral contraceptive pills for a patient I had known for over two years. I had delivered her second child two years ago and her third child nine weeks before this visit. She was one of my favorite patients, and I especially enjoyed treating her and her children.

After her second delivery, this 26-year-old black woman began having financial and marital difficulties and wanted to use a form of birth control. I instructed her to return to the office for a six-week postpartum examination or sooner if she had a menstrual period. She returned at six weeks postpartum stating that she had bled slightly for two days one week after delivery, but had not had a period since that time. I gave her three sample birth control packs and instructed her to begin the first pack of pills on the fifth day of her next menstrual cycle and to see me in three to four months for reevaluation. She never began the birth control pills but again became pregnant shortly before her husband left her and the two children. She returned to the office two months later to confirm her third pregnancy. The prenatal course, labor, and delivery went surprisingly well. Four weeks postpartum she was started on birth control pills and returned for this visit five weeks later.

The Incident

To my surprise, the first thing I noticed on entering the examination room was the patient's nine-week-old son lying on her lap with his right arm bandaged in an elastic brace. It was the first time I had learned of his fractured right humerus, which occurred 13 days earlier and was treated by one of my partners. According to the note in her son's chart, he "started to fall off his bed and his mother caught him by his right arm." Two days later his right arm was "swollen below the shoulder and he cried whenever he moved it so she brought him to our office for evaluation." I was not working in the center that day so my partner examined the patient, diagnosed the spiral fracture, padded and splinted the arm in an appropriate manner, and scheduled him to be reevaluated by me in one week. He also notified the county social service agency of the incident as is required by law for cases of suspected child abuse.

At first I felt embarrassed and guilty that I was seeing the mother and knew nothing about her son's injury. I was also angry at my partner for not telling me about the incident. More important, though, I was concerned that a woman who seemed loving and caring toward her three children was going to be labeled as a child abuser. Her children were always well-dressed despite her lack of resources.

I asked her what had happened and she reported the incident as my partner had described. She was not upset that a social worker interviewed her about possible child neglect, but admitted that she needed some time away from the children and didn't know how to accomplish it. She was receptive to several strategies suggested by our nurse specialist and me. We proposed that she arrange for at least one day per week to engage in an enjoyable activity without the children as well as to investigate job opportunities through the Comprehensive Employment and Training Act.

Discussion

I consider myself the family physician for this patient and her children, but several events disrupted my impression of our relationship. First, I still feel guilty that I erred in prescribing birth control pills too late to prevent a third pregnancy at a time when this patient was already under considerable stress from marital and financial difficulties. Second, I was angry at my partner for not informing me about an important new problem with one of my families. Third, I feel ambivalent about labeling someone as a child abuser, especially someone who demonstrated loving and caring parental skills toward her children.

This case has made me aware of several issues: (1) How do family physicians resolve errors they feel they make with patients? My colleagues reassure me that I did everything that I could and that preventing a third pregnancy was not completely within my control. Colleagues, however, tend to be overly supportive at these times and I still feel responsible. (2) What is the best way to communicate about patients we see for our partners? (3) How do we resolve the dilemma of knowing and liking a patient and reporting that person to outside authorities? In this case I feel that there were circumstances I knew of which others might not understand or consider in dealing with my patient. My knowledge of the patient allowed me to take advantage of the mother's caring skills in order to devise a remedial plan for her and consequently for her children. Am I too protective of my patients? I ask myself, if I had been in the office to treat the fracture, would I have reported her to the child abuse agency?

Commentary

The physician in the case presented raises three issues: (1) how to deal with the ambivalent feelings we have when we are faced with a decision to report a patient, in this case a suspected child abuser, to a social agency; (2) how physicians in a group practice setting should communicate about serious problems they encounter when covering for their colleagues; and (3) how to handle personal guilt over real or perceived errors we make in our care of patients.

That this mother should be reported to a social service agency as a suspected child abuser should not be open to question. The injury was an unusual and serious one for which the mother's accident description was questionable. The mother admitted that she was under stress and that she needed time away from her children. Additionally, several other risk factors for child abuse were present, including a single parent family, the addition of an unplanned third child, and an economically stressed family. These factors should compel any physician to suspect abuse, and it is only the suspicion, rather than the certainty of abuse, which doctors in all 50 states are required to report. Since child abuse and neglect is now recognized as the leading cause of death in children in the United States, the medical profession needs to err on the side of reporting rather than overlooking suspected child abuse cases. It is useful for a physician in a group to share concern over making such a referral to an agency with his professional colleagues. The collective opinion of the group will usually overcome the reticence of an individual physician, especially if the hesitancy to report is built on the physician's guilt over management or fear of damaging a relationship with an individual patient. The sharing of responsibility for a difficult decision by a group can be used positively by the primary physician in explaining this decision to the patient. Additionally, referral to such an agency realistically should be viewed as a way of helping rather than punishing a stressed parent.

The physician's partner, however, should not have been the one to make the referral to the social service agency if the primary physician was available to do so within a reasonable period of time. This is the second issue raised by the physician involved in this incident. Most group practices (consisting of more than one physician provider) have worked out methods of communicating about patients seen for their colleagues. This process is taught in most family practice residency programs. Methods used include routing patient charts seen by an alternative provider to the primary provider before they are refiled, utilizing a cover slip detailing the name of the patient seen, the problem for which he or she was seen, and the alternate provider's disposition of the problem. If the absence of the primary provider would keep charts out of circulation too long, the line listing alone can be circulated, frequently in conjunction with a listing of phone messages handled for the primary provider. In addition, conferences at weekly (or some other appropriate) intervals may be scheduled to discuss patients whose care has involved more than one physician. These discussions should be held on a regularly occurring, regularly scheduled basis. Still other groups of family physicians have made the physician's nurse or some other member of the health care team responsible for communicating about patients seen by alternate providers. Any system of communication, however, should be utilized for the briefest coverage and for routine problems as well as for more serious problems.

The final issue raised by the physician is the most complex. How do physicians deal with guilt they experience when they feel they have made an error in management? Important here is the feeling that they have made an error. No one who reads this incident would conclude that this physician made any error, and we learn that this indeed was also the conclusion of his clinical colleagues when he discussed his management with them. However, he still feels responsible. An unpublished survey of 57 graduates of our family practice residency program showed that concern over patient management caused significant or moderate stress in 86 percent of these physicians. Generally, it is safe to assume that most physicians at some time experience stress concerning the management of patients. Little attention has been paid in training programs to this form of stress. Physicians seek to dissipate their concern by formal consultation or informal communication with colleagues. However, as in this case, guilt over perceived errors in management may not be significantly lessened in this way. After discussing the case with colleagues, if it is acceptable from a medicolegal perspective, it may help to discuss concern with the patient involved. The patient's perception of the care received may be totally different from that of the provider. Often when the physician understands more fully how the patient feels about the quality of care, it may either allay concern or help focus concern in a more constructive manner. Finally, in cases where a physician's guilt still remains high, professional counseling for the physician may be needed and should be sought.

David M. Holden, M.D.
Professor of Family Medicine and Pediatrics
Director, Wesley Medical Center Family Practice Residency Program
University of Kansas School of Medicine
Wichita, Kansas

Commentary

When faced with having made errors in the care of patients, it is important that the doctor's self-esteem be based, not upon having been perfect, but rather upon doing the best he can. If the individual is so inflexible as not to be able to accept an error, he will have a great deal of difficulty in any profession requiring technical skill and judgment made without an absolute idea of potential outcome.

The author of this particular critical incident seems to have a tendency to be overly concerned about errors. It certainly is important that one avoid making errors, learn from them, and feel bad for having made them, but not "whip" oneself for errors or take full blame when involvement was merely contributory. The person most responsible for the patient's behavior is the patient herself. The physician should not adopt a feeling of full responsibility for the course of patients' lives since he is not the one ultimately responsible in a management sense. Certainly, sometimes patients' lives are in the doctor's hands, but still the physician is not responsible for the order of the patients' lives. The physician's dwelling over a past behavior won't help the patient and demonstrates a particular obsessiveness which could become a problem if it has not already. If the physician wants to help this patient now, given the present situation, it is important to make sure that he is available to the patient when she is in a crisis regarding this infant or any of her other children. If he cannot be available, he should help her find someone whom she can call so that she won't abuse her child in the future. Since the author seems to already have a good relationship with the patient, it would be desirable if he could be the one the patient could call in times of crisis.

As for the best way to communicate about patients seen for partners, the incident does not make clear what communicative pathways were utilized. It was stated that such was noted in the boy's chart, but it is not known whether that was part of a family chart. Realistically, many try to make a special attempt to communicate what seems to be extra-important, but often we fail. The issue here seems to be not just the breakdown of communication but also the feelings toward the partner regarding his not communicating the important information. What is potentially more essential is that the primary physician did not communicate his disappointment, irritation, or anger to his partner for not previously sharing the information. The encouragement of mutual communication is advisable, and if a partner is unable to handle irritation that is directed at him, then he may not be the most suitable partner.

It is a dilemma to know and like a patient and have to report a suspected child abuse to authorities. While one may not always like the reporting law, society as a whole has judged that child abuse must always be reported, and that stand should not be turned aside lightly. The doctor in the critical incident seems to make a frequent perceptive error that because the children seem well cared for in terms of hygiene and clothing, and because the mother is personable, she wouldn't be seriously abusive. Facts do not support this position. It is best to tell the parent who is suspected of child abuse that he or she is still liked and, although one feels bad in doing so, the incident must be reported. Often patients stay with the physician even though he has reported them. Abusive parents often can fool the physician because they have a good ability to meet the needs of a parental figure. They have grown up in a parent-oriented family where children are expected to care for their siblings (Kempe & Helfer, 1972) so they know how to take care of those in authority and they can be very pleasant, nice, and cooperative to parent figures while abusing their children.

With regard to feeling guilty about the patient becoming pregnant, it would perhaps assuage feelings of guilt if the physician let the patient know that he felt bad about what happened. It seems legally inadvisable to admit guilt particularly in this case when there is no evidence that the doctor committed any action suggestive of malpractice. To further deal with the feeling of guilt, the doctor might find an older colleague who would be willing to act as a sounding board. Many physicians have difficulty confessing to their peers because they are in competition with them. In addition, doctors have difficulty confessing to other than fellow professionals because of fear of lawsuits or a feeling someone outside the profession would not understand. Perhaps an older, experienced professional would provide a kindly support. It's important for everyone to have a confidant, particularly people who are under such stressful and demanding working conditions as physicians.

The outcome of the handling of the incident appears to be correct. The case was reported. The parent was supported and was aided in finding alternate activities. It seems appropriate for the doctor to communicate with the partner about his feelings and to work out a better communication system. It is also advisable to have some psychological "work" regarding feelings of responsibility and guilt.

I think many physicians become aloof from their patients as a way of handling their feeling of guilt and sadness about a patient's physical discomfort or about their life-threatening illness. The distancing results in more unresolved feelings of guilt, and this can cause yet further distancing from their patients. While an admission of error seems legally dangerous and an invitation to a malpractice suit, a physician can express to a patient his concern for the patient, his sorrow that the patient is suffering, and his empathy for the patient. Letting a patient know that you feel bad when they feel bad or are in pain or are depressed seems to be a good medical practice. A necessary resource is a colleague, friend, or loved one readily available to discuss feelings in a constructive and helpful way. This will help to avoid burying feelings and distancing self from patients.

Another issue is that of interpersonal communication with colleagues. Communication takes time. Many physicians do not have a great deal of spare time so they tend not to communicate. Many are also psychologically isolated professionals, either because of their own personal needs and vulnerabilities or because they have tended to wall themselves off from everyone because of the painful experiences endured and witnessed every day. Briefly, I urge physicians to risk being more open about their feelings, for an emotionally constricted life is not a life which feels full or rewarding. Many of the people doctors fear to communicate with because of feeling vulnerable would be delighted to share in a mutual communication and sharing of feelings.

Also an issue is the need for better education about child abuse. State laws requiring that suspected cases of child abuse be reported also protect doctors from malpractice when they are acting with good intent. The physician in the incident seems fairly naive about child abuse. He seems not to realize that a patient can look competent and can love his or her children but still be physically abusive. I would suggest a number of articles on child abuse as a first step toward self-education. Many communities have hospital or community child protection teams which can provide expert assistance in dealing with child abuse cases. In addition, one can become familiar with the social service system in the area to provide psychosocial support for the parent. Many communities also have an information and referral center which can be called upon by parents and professionals. These centers can provide information as to available services in the community. However, many patients are easily intimidated by the system and need continued encouragement. What the physician can do for parents is to help provide the needed support systems so that when there is a crisis, they will not react to the stress by physically abusing their children.

Resolution of these issues requires self-knowledge and psychological self-examination as well as communicative effort and ability. The issues are uncomfortable and therefore easy to put off, especially when there are more immediate, pressing activities to address. Failure to confront these issues, in the long run, can be costly. In the present case, nonresolution of the issues could result in a physician burdened with excessive and unnecessary guilt, a deteriorated relationship with a colleague and a patient, continuing child abuse by the patient, and the breaking of child abuse laws by a physician.

Alan L. Evans, Ph.D.
Clinical Psychologist
The Toledo Hospital
Toledo, Ohio

Reference

Kempe, C. H., & Helfer, R. E. *Helping the battered child and his family*. Philadelphia: Lippincott, 1972.

Suggested Reading

Evans, A. L. *Personality characteristics and disciplinary attitudes of child abusing mothers*. Saratoga, California: Century 21 Publishing Co., 1981.

30 / A Social Disease

An "Acid Test" for the Physician-Family
Relationship

Background

For the past 15 years, I have practiced in a rural community of 3,000 people. As is frequently the case in small towns, the physician becomes friends with many of his patients, causing problems of role contamination—doctor/friend—with resultant increased emotional involvement.

One couple, Roger and Jane, had become close friends of my wife and me. I had delivered their second and third children, taken out the tonsils and adenoids of one of their other children, treated the husband for a fractured ankle, and cared for their parents when they became ill while visiting. This past winter my wife and I went on a skiing trip with them and had an excellent vacation.

The Incident

Four months ago, Jane came to the office for her routine, yearly breast and pelvic exam and to renew her oral contraceptive. She stated that she had been in good health, with no symptoms or complications of the medication, and had been having regular periods without any vaginal irritation or discharge. The examination was normal. Pap smear and a routine cervical culture were taken.

The pathology reports on my desk several mornings later indicated a normal Pap smear but, to my surprise, the test for gonorrhea was positive. My first reaction was that there must have been a lab error. I then became concerned as to what should be my next move. After considering the options, I called Jane and told her that one of her tests was inconclusive and should be repeated. She asked, "I don't have cancer, do I?" I quickly reassured her that that was not the case. Her following question was, "What is it then?" I told her that I would give a full explanation when she came in for the repeat examination and suggested that I should see her that afternoon or the next day.

I rehearsed many possible ways of explaining the situation to Jane. They all troubled me. I was concerned about the probable disease and its management. I was concerned about the effect this diagnosis might have on Jane and Roger's relationship. I was also concerned about its possible effect on my professional and personal relationship with the family.

At that next visit, I informed her that one of the tests indicated there might be an infection. I again asked her questions about discharge and irritation that she or her husband might have recently experienced. She again denied the existence of symptoms. I then told her that the first test for gonorrhea was positive. With this, she broke down and started crying. After the tears slowed down, she told me that the only way she could have contracted gonorrhea was from her husband. She was very angry but consented to a repeat culture. I then drew blood for a serology test, administered penicillin therapy, and asked her permission to discuss this matter with her husband. She said that was not necessary; she would take care of it. She promised to telephone me later that evening or the next morning.

The next morning Jane and Roger came to my office. It was a difficult conversation, not our usual good-natured, happy, friendly talk. Jane cried frequently as Roger, slowly, and with many sighs, told the following story. He said that three weeks before he was on a professional trip and was entertained by the manufacturing company with dinner, alcoholic drinks to excess, and sexual relationships with a female "secretary" from the organization. Roger said that this was "the first time" any such activity on his part had taken place. A few days later he noticed a urethral irritation and discharge. He did not discuss this with anyone nor did he seek medical treatment. He did have sexual intercourse with his wife.

Roger was examined, proper specimens taken, and medical treatment for the infection was given.

I suggested that if there was any problem in resolving the personal and marital aspects of this situation that they should contact me.

Since that time my wife and I have rarely seen Jane and Roger socially. My wife wonders why they abruptly broke off our friendship and why we are no longer invited to their home for parties. Professionally, I cannot discuss the critical medical incident with my wife. She feels that possibly we have done something, socially, to offend them. I wonder if I could have handled the matter in a different way. Was my personal demeanor or professional conduct offensive to them?

Discussion

How does one keep the proper professional objectivity and distance and yet deal with patients, who are also friends, in a friendly, caring way? Should a physician avoid forming friendships with his patients? When patients who are personal friends respond to therapy, it is professionally and personally rewarding. However, when the results are not optimal, the resultant pain is also doubled.

Commentary

The situation described is certainly not uncommon, especially in rural practice. As every family physician with some practice time and experience knows, there are a number of ways, many of them less than satisfactory, to handle problems such as this.

In approaching either presenting partner, I am usually noncommital about a specific etiological agent until I'm fairly sure of the entire situation. I like to use general terms such as "infection" and bring the other partner in for necessary studies and probing conversation. Even in these enlightened days, many people are unaware of the variety and manifestations of the various sexually transmitted diseases and tend to accept the investigative process as a matter of fact. Of course, if stress is observed in one of the partners, this can be used as an opportunity for an open-ended question such as "How do you think you contracted this?" Also, the use of a statement as "sometimes this is transmitted by intercourse" can lead to an opening for discussion of extramarital contacts. This applies to the male more than to the female. The process of ventilation occurs when a patient has confidence both in the skills of a physician and in the physician's reputation in the community for absolutely protecting the confidentiality of each and every patient. This does not mean that the physician must be close-mouthed and perpetually withdrawn, but indicates the ability to parry personal inquiries about a patient with broad and noncompromising answers which do not disclose information of a personal nature or offend the questioner. At times, with repeated nosiness, a blunt response is all that is effective.

Physicians for years have practiced medicine for patients who in other settings are close personal friends without getting the two situations enmeshed. The basis for this is rigorous self-discipline on the part of the physician. Preparation for this begins in medical school by exposure to role models who can demonstrate this attitude. This development continues in residency programs through discussions with the attending staff and colleagues. Once in practice, establishing a relationship with a more experienced practitioner is of great benefit when situations such as that under discussion arise. Discussing possible courses of action with an experienced physician can be most reassuring and often leads to a reasonable solution.

In an urban practice, it may be possible for a physician to be completely isolated from social contact with his patients, but not likely. In a rural practice, it is almost impossible for a physician not to interact socially with this patients, especially over a period of time. Meeting patients as friends and co-workers in church, service clubs, children's school activities, sporting events such as hunting, fishing, and skiing opens many possibilities for filing away facts and impressions about people for later use when the physician–patient relationship is brought into play. In my opinion, such associations are highly desirable in that the more a physician knows about a sick or injured person the better the physician is able to be of assistance to that particular person. I do not mean that a physician must be socially close with every patient in the practice. This is obviously impossible and undesirable. The implication is that the physician, especially the family physician, must be aware of the needs of patients, their capability to help themselves, and activities within the community which may impact upon a particular situation.

In the critical incident under discussion I would have advised Jane that she had an infection of the cervix which needed to be treated. At the same time I would have informed her that sometimes these infections are passed between husband and wife and asked her to make an appointment for Roger to get some studies as well. At the time of Roger's visit, if he were a friend of mine, the information about the business trip would have surfaced and, depending upon his attitude, he would be offered several options, after appropriate treatment. The first of these options would be, particularly if this were a very stable marriage, for Roger to explain the situation to Jane, and if additional counseling were needed, I would offer to help. Another approach, particularly if Roger did not feel that his marriage could stand the stress of admission, would be to couch the diagnosis in general terms and avoid causing further difficulties between the two. Roger would also be thoroughly counseled about his activities on future business trips, including advice about use of the condom and personal hygiene should he expect to be involved in extramarital sexual activities in the future. The two cases of gonorrhea would have been reported to the Public Health Department as properly diagnosed and treated on the appropriate reporting form. In an incident such as this, I would advise the Health Department that I had performed the necessary epidemiological investigation and that no further effort on their part was necessary. Follow-up cultures and serologies would have been performed at the proper times, and my demeanor as well as that of my office staff would have been such that neither Roger nor Jane would have felt ashamed, afraid, or threatened.

Our social activity would have continued as before, again without innuendos on my part to Roger in front of or away from Jane. My wife would be totally unaware of the specifics of the illness or even of the visits to my office unless it was mentioned by Roger or Jane in routine conversation. A physician can care for people professionally and enjoy their friendship socially to everyone's advantage. In my own practice, situations such as the one discussed have occurred on a number of occasions. Proper management has been given without disruption of the marital unit, and friendly relations exist between members of my family and members of theirs to this day.

Sam A. Nixon, M.D.
Professor
Department of Family Practice
The University of Texas Medical School at Houston
Houston, Texas

Commentary

The contributor of this incident raises some important questions that unfortunately have no simple answers. An inherent difficulty would seem to exist when one tries to combine two differing kinds of relationships between the same individuals. While the problem in reporting the gonorrhea to the wife would have been difficult under any circumstances, the personal relationship with the couple and the physician's own feelings about this would tend to complicate the situation even further. Avoiding friendships with patients certainly could be one solution to this problem, but this may not be a realistic solution for the physician who is practicing in a rural or isolated setting. The physician's own personal and social needs might well be sacrificed to maintain this otherwise desirable separation of roles.

Some anticipation of this as a problem might be useful when a physician either becomes socially involved with patients or takes on new patients who are already friends. There may be a recognition with the patient/friend at the beginning of the dual relationship that it could get awkward for both of them. An awareness of this fact by both the physician and the patient might allow them to consider more carefully whether they would want to enter into this dual relationship. Certainly if the relationship becomes intense enough that the physician's judgment could not remain objective enough to be therapeutic, then the physician himself/herself would have the obligation to withdraw from one aspect of the dual relationship. The physician's handling of this difficult issue seemed to be basically sound; however, there are some areas where another approach might have been considered. For example, when the physician phoned the wife asking her to come in to repeat the test, his vagueness in an attempt to be evasive led to needless worry by the wife that she might have cancer. While it was well that he reassured her on the telephone, some other approach might have prevented this needless worry. It may be that the physician decided it was better to take the chance on this needless worry rather than convey some very disturbing news to the wife over the telephone. A more significant alteration in strategy might have been considered by the physician with regard to his follow-up. He had treated their medical problem and offered to meet with the couple again for help in resolving the personal and marital aspects of the situation. I would particularly have supported his giving them a referral for a marriage counselor in a nearby community if they desired to use it. It might have been possible, however, for him to have scheduled a recheck appointment a few weeks following this last reported contact. While the specific medical treatment of their condition may not have required it, the broader treatment of these patients, which would include their emotional well-being, might suggest that a recheck on their emotional state and relationship would be appropriate. However, it may be at this particular point that the physician backed off from his professional role and was influenced by his friendship role. One might raise the hypothetical question of whether or not the physician might have scheduled some follow-up contact with the couple if he had not been friendly with them. The question is whether the physician's own discomfort and embarrassment for his friends interfered with his optimal management of their care. By being aware of the global aspects of his treatment, which include the emotional as well as the physical, a more aggressive consideration of their status and relationship might have been indicated.

In approaching it from the opposite perspective, it is possible that the physician's objectivity interfered with his reaching out to his friends as friends. One might anticipate that embarrassment was a factor in the severed social relationship between the physician and the couple. Reaching out to them either individually or as a couple might have been indicated on that basis, along with a clear statement to them that his awareness of the incident would not affect his caring for them as a couple or his wanting to be their friend. In addition, an explicit statement that, of course, his wife would not know about the incident might have been reassuring. While patients may understand the medical ethics involved in maintaining confidentiality, specific reassurance about this point might have been helpful to the couple.

The larger issue raised by this incident involves the dual relationships that may occur between physicians and patients, particularly in smaller communities. The possible social isolation a physician might impose upon himself/herself to avoid this conflict would seem to be another aspect of this issue. The concept of optimal balance has been used in dealing with helping relationships. On the one hand, the helper (in this case the physician) cannot appear too remote or cold if he or she wants to be helpful. On the other hand, a relationship that is too close and overly involved also has dangers of not being helpful. To maintain this optimal relationship in social relationships may require a delicate balance on the part of the physician. If the physician had a colleague with whom he might discuss such difficult issues, some of the burden might be lifted. One of the problems for the physician in a small community includes the professional isolation that would include lack of opportunity to talk out professional issues and receive some peer reactions and support without a breach of professional ethics. A remedy for the optimal-social-distance dilemma for the physician in a small town might well include then a professional colleague, possibly in a neighboring town, with whom the physician could talk out some of these difficult situations.

Denis J. Lynch, Ph.D.
Associate Professor
Department of Family Medicine
Medical College of Ohio at Toledo
Toledo, Ohio

31 / Time Invaders
Patient Demands and Time Off

Background

I was relaxing one night at a family party which involved my daughter and her new fiance. The laughter and festive mood were interrupted by a ringing telephone which my wife answered, since I was not on call. Being a small-town physician with limited uninterrupted hours for personal and family involvement, the telephone has frequently been regarded by me and my family as one of the worst inventions ever created.

The Incident

One of our family's close social friends was calling to request medical care for his mother, who was a patient of mine. He knew that I was not on call, having been told by the answering service, which had instructed him to call my partner. Many of our friends have our unlisted phone number in order to call various members of the family for social reasons. Tom asked that my wife call me to the phone, and then he insisted that I attend to his mother, who he felt was seriously ill.

I felt angry that he had broken our established protocol and invaded my private life. I tried to explain that my partner was available to treat his mother and that I would prefer that he call him. He refused, and I offered to call my partner and give him the message and his phone number. He reluctantly accepted this proposal.

The mother did have a small stroke and was hospitalized. The next morning, when I was on call, I saw her on hospital rounds. Tom and his wife were present and I discussed with them their mother's condition. Neither of us discussed the previous evening's incident. I felt frustrated and guilty that I had to protect my private time. I felt resentful that they had used my friendship. I also felt guilty that I did not accept the call to take care of their mother during a serious illness.

This is not the first time this problem has occurred with this couple.

Discussion

I have found it difficult to insulate my professional and personal life. In a small town, a physician is highly visible during his "off hours." Is it necessary to leave town to become unavailable? Is it necessary for family members to lie and say, "He is not in"?

On various occasions I have discussed this matter with friends and neighbors. I have found it difficult and frequently the individual becomes offended.

Commentary

This incident, which involved the "invasion" of the off call time of a small-town family physician and the feelings which this generated in him, is well known to most physicians who have functioned in such a setting. This represents a common conflict between patient demands or patient perception of the role of a physician and the physician's perception of that same role. The availability of time for self and for family hinges upon the physician's attitude concerning this incident, as does the physician's satisfaction with small-town practice. Thus, consideration of this type of incident and its implications should be done by any physician before embarking on medical practice in a small community.

The role of the small-town physician, as perceived by his patients, differs from that of his colleagues in the large city, the most important difference stemming from the fact that the small-town physician's social contacts will be drawn almost exclusively from his cohort of patients. The two roles, doctor in the office and neighbor at home, cannot be separated entirely, and expectations that they will be are unrealistic.

Additionally, the knowledge which most small-town inhabitants have about their friends and neighbors (including the doctor) is considerable. Family living habits, activities of the children, and external evidence of affluence are quite likely to be known to some extent by the public consisting of patient-social friends. The role of a community physician may well make his personal life of greater interest than is true for other vocations. The "glass house" phenomenon is usually a reality for the small-town physician.

These facts, coupled with a public attitude that equates physician knowledge of patient health problems with physician concern about these problems, create a framework within which the physician will live and work. The public expectation is that the "caring" qualities of the physician punch no time clock. Added to the pressures that this expectation can generate are those produced by the physician's own compulsions and insecurities. Guilt and frustration with their resultant unhappiness and anxiety are always a possibility.

Thus, before embarking on a small-town practice, it would seem wise for the physician to come to grips with the fact that he will be expected to function more in the realm of quasi-community property than might be true in the city. The degree to which this can be changed is limited and when accomplished is usually the result of long-term "practice education." The physician who would insist upon total separation of medical activities from his social and personal life might be well advised to locate in a more heavily populated area where relative anonymity can be achieved.

Lest it be interpreted that there is no virtue in being a small-town physician, it must be stated that for many of us the above-discussed sacrifices are more than outweighed by the warmth of the close relationships, the satisfaction gained by being a surrogate member of many families, the freedom to practice family medicine in its fullest sense, and the advantages of raising a family in a small community. It must be noted that for almost one-half of the graduates of family practice residency programs these factors hold sway.

The alternatives which the physician in this incident had when his special free time was interrupted might be examined to see whether there were any avenues of action available to him which might have allowed him to "have his cake and eat it, too."

1. Leave the phone unanswered during time off. This is difficult for a physician. The call might be from his partner, from an absent family member, or from some other desired contact. Since he is probably known to be home, this option might well result in the anxious son arriving at the front door. The uneasiness produced by an unanswered phone is not conducive to a relaxed and comfortable evening. This does not appear to be a satisfactory solution.

2. Have a wife or child answer the phone and state that the physician is not available. This can easily make the person answering the phone uncomfortable and place that person in the position of having to evaluate the degree of an emergency. Hedging or prevaricating about the availability of the physician is difficult for family members, questionable training for children, and likely to be productive of guilt for the entire family.

3. The phone could be answered by the physician, who requests that the partner be called. This was the avenue chosen in this incident with the somewhat unsatisfactory results described.

4. The phone could be answered by the physician, who makes an immediate house call if patient is not agreeable to calling the partner. All things considered, this might have been the most satisfactory answer. Distances in small towns are short, as is travel time. Assessment of the patient can be done and plans for care formulated, usually within a very brief time. Then the physician can indicate that he will call the partner concerning the problem and plans, and the partner can assume temporary care until the following day. This approach leaves the patient and family satisfied with minimal disruption of the physician's program since often a half-hour or less is required to do this. It does not generate feelings of guilt in the physician and rarely deprives him of significant time with his family. This also can serve as a first educational step for the demanding patient who is brought to the realization that the physician, while genuinely caring, has both a personal life and confidence in his partner. It might also be noted that this helps to maintain the desired image of the physician's role within his family. Such departures from family social gatherings are unquestionably beneficial in building a practice.

There are several other facts about this incident worthy of comment. First, the possession of an unlisted phone number by a small-town physician is likely to be both futile and inconvenient for the physician and the family. Inability to contact the physician by phone will certainly increase the incidence of visits to the physician's home by patients. This may be inappropriate for the provision of needed care and inconvenient to family activities. If the physician chooses to insist on his right to free time, he will find that this is more difficult to handle than it would be over the telephone and also more productive of feelings of guilt.

Second, the fact that the physician purposefully avoided talking about what to him was an emotionally charged topic when seeing his patient the following morning is significant and indicates an inability to bring the conflict to a satisfactory resolution. He may find that this interferes with his attitude about and treatment of this patient during the hospitalization. This could have been an appropriate time for education of the patient's family about the physician's "system" of care and the partnership arrangement. His inability to broach the matter lost him this opportunity.

The physician states that it is difficult to separate his professional and personal life. In a small town this may well be a practical impossibility since the color and the make of his car are known, as are the barber he goes to, the bank he utilizes, his usual golf dates or fishing holes, and his favorite restaurant. Even the police force is likely to join in this conspiracy against his off hours if an emergency arises—cruising the community until the doctor is found! The physician might well consider that he or his family might have utilized their own friendships of others, such as the plumber, TV repairman, or auto mechanic by requesting after hours or weekend help. It's likely they have. He should remember this.

Genuine family medicine as practiced in a small town is a hard taskmaster with demands that at times are determined only by the patient's perception of a health problem, which often ignores the time or date. In the broad sense, a segment of the community—his patients—constitutes the physician's "family" with all the obligations and rewards which this implies. The community will place the physician on a pedestal regardless of his desire or intent. Its ultimate configuration will be of his making.

James G. Price, M.D.
Associate Professor
Department of Family Practice
University of Kansas
Kansas City, Kansas

Commentary

The answer to both questions asked by the physician who describes this incident is no. It is not only unnecessary but not possible for a physician to leave town every time he wants to spend an evening quietly with his family. Furthermore, in answer to his second question, he would lose credibility quickly with other physicians and patients alike if he lies and states that he is not in when in reality he is in and available. He has handled the incident behaviorally quite well, but has apparently considerable difficulty with his feelings about this incident. In my commentary I wish to deal first with his feelings about this incident and later to consider alternative ways of handling the incident.

The author of the incident states that he felt angry that his friend insisted that he take time away from his family when he had arranged for someone else to take his calls. Being placed in the personally vulnerable position of being asked to attend to the friend's mother at the same time the physician has obligations to his own family places him on the horns of a dilemma for which there is no solution. He felt angry that his friend had invaded his private life and had demanded that he leave his family. He may have felt further frustration and anger because there was no solution to the predicament in which his friend placed him. To meet this demand would cause considerable emotional discomfort and at the same time to deny it caused discomfort.

This is an unavoidable situation for the physician in this incident because he is a small-town physician in great demand with limited hours for personal and family involvement. Even so, it is absolutely essential that he reserve time which he can devote to activities which are gratifying to himself, whether that time be spent with his family or in some other pursuit. Each individual, particularly a physician, must carefully guard against being overwhelmed by demands placed on him by other people. The impact of his and his family's reaction to those demands are made clear by his statement that "the telephone has frequently been regarded by me and my family as one of the worst inventions ever created." The telephone usually brings the first communication of a demand which will be made on the physician. Whatever amount of time agreed upon by the physician and his family as the minimum which they must have in order to be reasonably happy as a family, as well as the time needed by the physician himself to restore the emotional and physical energy and strength to replace the drains created by his work, must be set aside and guarded religiously to prevent emotional and physical illness and serious personal and family problems. Each individual's and family's requirements differ in this respect. It can be determined prior to a physician setting up practice, but usually it is determined by trial and error over time with the physician or his family developing physical or sociopsychological symptoms prior to his limiting the time that he devotes to his practice. Once this minimal time and energy requirement is known, it must be regarded by the physician and his family and his colleagues as the highest priority of his many commitments.

In order for the physician to avoid feeling angry when others make demands on this extremely important time which he and his family have set aside, he must first accept as a fact that there will be continued demands made on that time merely because of the situation in which he lives. Then he must accept the fact that there are limitations to the amount of energy which he can devote to his practice and a limit to his commitment to his friends. He cannot avoid coming to grips with the internal conflicts produced by his sense of duty and his anger regarding the demands made on him. Once he confronts himself with the options and chooses that option most rational, the conflict is minimized.

To paraphrase his statements, the doctor felt resentful, guilty, and frustrated because of the position his friend had put him in and because he had not responded to the call of duty. Usually a strong conscience is helpful for a physician to provide good treatment for his patients and also for him to fulfill the role of physician and advisor to his patients. Yet if he is overly conscientious about meeting all demands made on him, he will not be able to survive as a small-town physician. He must consult his own conscience with the agreed-upon limitations of his own personal needs and his family's needs. He may ease his guilt, resentment, frustration, and anger over time as he comes to believe, not only intellectually, but emotionally, that there is a relatively specific limit to his ability to meet the demands of his practice. He must also invest himself in his family and ultimately reserve time for the rest and relaxation which will help to restore and rebuild the emotional and physical strength to cope adequately with his work as a physician.

To assume that his patients, other physicians, or other people in his community will stop making demands merely because he has another physician covering for him is unrealistic. He must accept the fact that they will continue to make demands but that he can gain greater comfort while being less disturbed by those demands.

There are alternatives to the behaviors which he elected on the evening of the incident. (1) For example, his wife might have told his friend that his family has adopted the policy that there will be no business on his evenings off. (2) The author might have attended the friend's mother on request. (3) Even the personal phone can be attached to an automatic answering device which merely instructs all calls to go to his partner. In the case of personal calls, they could be screened by the partner. (4) He could take the phone off the hook. However, none of these behaviors or any others that the reader might suggest will avoid the internal feelings regarding the incident as described by the author. He must come to grips internally with the feelings generated by such an incident and must think through the priorities as described above and come to some form of internal peace regarding conflicts produced by such incidents as a solution to the problem, rather than finding a solution through the manipulation of the people involved or the demands which they have made.

All physicians need to take heed that they provide excellent service and meet the needs of their communities to a practicable extent, lest they find themselves alone without patients and friends. Yet they must not hurt themselves or their families by overcompliance to demands. This physician can take solace in his being a person who is needed in his community. There must be a balance between what he gives to his society and what he saves for himself.

John P. Kemph, M.D.
Vice President for Academic Affairs
Dean of the School of Medicine
Medical College of Ohio at Toledo
Toledo, Ohio

32 / Past Due
Nonpayment of Fees

Background

Mr. A. was probably a living example of Willie Loman of *Death of a Salesman* fame. He had worked hard all his life and tried to participate in the best way he could with his rather domineering, very forceful wife in the rearing of their four children. It seemed as the years went by that he would go from job to job, sales position to sales position, but he had trouble being financially successful. Nevertheless, his family managed well enough, with children going to work at early ages, yet becoming very well-educated and cultured. His account at the office would always be one of those to come across my desk month after month as being either unpaid or having a balance that was growing larger instead of smaller even with an occasional monthly payment being made. Quite different from other families with delinquent accounts was the reaction of Mr. A's wife, who would always respond to an overdue notice by becoming quite incensed and angry. She would make sarcastic remarks either in writing or verbally to the office personnel who would attempt to secure an occasional payment on the account. "What to do" with this family and account was always a monthly problem for me.

The Incident

Mr. A. was in the office and was quite excited. He had recovered from the triple bypass surgery done six months previously and was feeling good. His blood sugars were under good control with his dosage of insulin, although he was having difficulty following his diet. His excitement stemmed from the fact that he had just been notified that he was going to get a job that he had been trying to get for over a year. This was an executive position with a large national company and would, in fact, be a realization of a lifetime dream. "Do you think I can make it physically, Doc?" Mr. A asked me with obvious anxiety in his face and eyes. I reassured him that I thought he could.

What followed over the ensuing several months seemed like a nightmare. Mr. A. developed chest pains and severe hypoglycemic reactions with apparently normal blood sugars. There were many visits to the emergency room and several hospitalizations with many cardiac and other medical subspecialty consultations. Yes, we all agreed that he did have coronary heart disease and diabetes, but these certainly did not account for all of his symptoms. Finally, due to absence from work because of illness, the company that had just hired him to a dream job fired him.

His past-due account at the office grew logarithmically. No payments were made and, in fact, the insurance payments that should have come to me managed to get into his hands and, you guessed it, I never saw a dollar. I finally had a conversation with him and suggested an excellent medical source for him at the Veterans Administration Clinic. We had, in fact, filled out some 15 insurance forms and repeated questionnaires concerning his disability and helped him in applying for many different kinds of benefits. When it came time to make the big decision about turning this account over for collection, I decided to cancel the account and wrote Mr. A. a letter wishing him well and telling him that he did not owe me anything. Several months later it became apparent that Mr. A. again had some source of income and was seeking medical care elsewhere. There was an ill-feeling between his family and me, their "ex-physician."

Background

Mrs. B. was one of the best operators that the Bell System ever hired. She was extremely competent on her job and was making advancements rapidly. She had been my patient since before she was married. As her personal physician I had gone through marriage, two deliveries, and times of sorrow and happiness with her. Over the years it became apparent that Mrs. B. was having trouble keeping up with the payments on her expanding account. She would make payments, but about the time that she would start to reduce the total balance, one or more of the children would get sick or her diabetic husband would get into trouble because of excessive drinking. Her husband, unlike Mrs. B., had trouble holding a job. He had tried many different jobs from sales to laboring and finally had a job that lasted some time as a stevedore. Because he was constantly getting into trouble, it became apparent that the marriage was in great jeopardy. Finally, Mr. and Mrs. B. were divorced and one of the sons was caught stealing and sent to prison.

The Incident

After many conversations and letters, it became painfully necessary to turn the account over for collection. Mr. B. ended up in a hospital in another city and paid the collector only after legal steps were taken. Approximately one year later, Mrs. B. called and asked me if I would please accept her and her son again as patients. She offered to pay cash for all services rendered at the time they are rendered and yes, she still had her position as a telephone operator. I accepted her back into my practice with a warm feeling and my relationship with Mrs. B. and her son has been a very pleasant one ever since.

Discussion

The above two cases are examples of a frequent dilemma in which a physician finds himself with patients who cannot or will not pay their bills. In the case of Mr. A., the decision was not to send the bill to a collector and cancel the rather large sum that was owed. The results were rather ironic in that when the patient again became able to afford a physician, he and his family went elsewhere and never offered to repay the canceled amount and, as a matter of fact, have continued a feeling of ill-will. In the case of Mrs. B., on the other hand, the decision was made to turn over an account to a collector and, in this case, the patient and the family returned and we started out with a greater feeling of mutual respect for one another. I don't know the answer to this dilemma, and there is no single answer for every case. I believe that these cases represent an example of the uncertainty of results that one can expect with difficult collection cases.

Commentary

The contract between physician and patient involves negotiations that determine the relationship between two individuals, the constraints under which care will be rendered, and the mutual obligations of provider and recipient. Payment of the physician's fee is an important component of the medical contract and, in fact, patients often cite fees as a reason for complaints against physicians (Cooke, 1976; Kasteler, Kane, Olsen, & Thetford, 1976). In addition, payment or nonpayment of the physician's fee is one of the few avenues by which the patient can express his feelings regarding the health care experience. The incidents involving the A. and B. families are two instances in which fees were not paid promptly. In the case of the A. family, no payment was obtained at all. Mr. B. paid the collection agency only after legal steps were taken.

What is the significance of nonpayment? Inability of the family to pay the physician's fee must always be considered. Yet even in these instances, "medically indigent" individuals usually seem to find money not only for food and shelter, but often for tobacco, alcohol, and gasoline. Whether or not there are true financial problems, payment of the physician's fee is accorded a priority which will be influenced by both the relationship with the doctor and the significance of the fee to the patient and family.

Barnlund (1976) has explored the meaning of human illness as a symbolic as well as a physical condition. The difference between disease and illness lies in the psychosocial implications of biologic dysfunction—the integration of the disorder with its meaning for the patient. Some measure of this "meaning" is necessarily transferred to the physician's fee statement. Thus, even the most intellectually objective patient's response will be influenced by the ongoing doctor–patient relationship and failure to receive an anticipated explanation.

Of course, the optimum and desired response is the prompt payment of a fee. Happily most patients express satisfaction with their medical encounters, and fees are generally paid within a reasonable time (Charney, 1972). Payment or failure to pay a fee may be linked to certain aspects of the health care process. For example, in 800 outpatient visits reported by Francis, Korsch, and Morris (1969), key factors in satisfaction (and compliance) were the extent to which patient expectations were met, lack of warmth in the doctor–patient relationship, and failure to receive an anticipated explanation.

In many instances, the cause of nonpayment is obscure and represents "acting-out" behavior on the part of the patient. Anger, guilt, and blame may all play roles. Nonpayment of the physician's fee may be a transference reaction in which feelings concerning the illness are shifted to the physician. One common mechanism used by patients is denial: the patient (and family) deny the existence of alcoholism, obesity, or signs suggesting malignancy and, hence, also deny their financial obligation to the physician. Blame-setting can result in litigation as well as nonpayment of fees, as a disgruntled patient seeks ways in which physical misfortune can be ascribed to the physician's surgical ineptitude, diagnostic incompetence, or referral delay. If the physician can be blamed for the patient's current predicament, is it not justifiable to withhold fee payment?

The patients and families described in the critical incident seem plausible examples of inappropriate responses to the physician's fee statement. It appears that Mr. A. associates his physician's treatment with failure at work and, ultimately, life itself. After all, was not the physician dead wrong in his opinion that Mr. A. could "make it physically" on the dream job? Failure can only be the fault of the physician. Mrs. A.'s verbal abuse may merely be an extension of blame-seeking behavior within the family.

When the time came to finally take action concerning the A. family account, a referral to the Veterans Administration may have been interpreted as abandonment. I can almost hear Mr. A. thinking, "The doctor was wrong about my ability to return to work. Now when I need him most, he's dismissing me just because I'm a little behind on my bill." What's more, writing off the account assaulted Mr. A.'s self-respect, although such may have been a more prudent course than referring the account for collection. Nevertheless, Mr. (and probably Mrs.) A. almost certainly blamed the physician for their disappointment following an inaccurate prognosis regarding return to work and the ultimate dismissal from the practice. With such strong feelings of righteous indignation, this family feels justified in not paying the physician's bill.

The B. family probably represents some legitimate inability to pay, coupled with the husband's denial of his drinking and hence of his financial obligation to the physician. In this instance I suspect that the meaning the patient associated with the illness was projected to the fee statement. Nevertheless, a good relationship was maintained with Mrs. B. and her son. Why? Because the family physician met their expectations. He managed their medical problems confidently and treated them fairly. I am sure they perceived nothing unfair about the account being turned over for collection. Thus, when Mr. and Mrs. B. were divorced, a new physician–family contract was negotiated with a restatement of expectations which included how fees were to be paid.

These cases illustrate two of the many fee dilemmas faced by the practicing physician. What are some guidelines that can help assure rational and ethical responses to nonpayment of fees? First of all, physician, patient, and family must all be clear concerning their mutual expectations. The medical contract should be outlined at an early visit, including some discussion of fee payments. Fee statements should be presented openly, and the patient should be given every opportunity to pay when in the office. Each family's bill should be aged with reminders to indicate when an account is overdue and to alert the physician when a fee problem is developing.

When it becomes apparent that a payment problem exists, the physician should consider the following: What is the meaning of this bill to the patient? What illness does it concern and what feelings does it evoke for the individual and the family? Based upon knowledge of the family income and lifestyle, how is this statement likely to rank in their bill-paying priorities? Is there some acting-out behavior going on? Is the patient using nonpayment of the bill to express dissatisfaction, anger, or blame? What can the physician and the office staff do to help the patient meet his or her obligations?

The events related to medical fees receive insufficient attention in medical education and training. Most physicians lack full awareness of current fees for health care services. In addition, residents in training programs and indeed many practitioners are insulated from the problems patients face in paying bills. Yet fee payments and nonpayments represent a handy index of patients' opinions, feelings, and perceptions of the doctor–patient relationship. It would be appropriate for family physicans to initiate further study of this integral component of the physician–patient contract.

Robert B. Taylor, M.D.
Associate Professor
Department of Family and Community Medicine
Bowman Gray School of Medicine
Winston-Salem, North Carolina

References

Barnlund, D. C. The mystification of meaning: Doctor–patient encounters. *Journal of Medical Education,* 1976, *51,* 716–725.

Charney, E. Patient–doctor communication: Implications for the physician. *Pediatric Clinics of North America,* 1972, *19*(2), 263–279.

Cooke, C. L. Patient complaints against physicians in the Richmond area during 1973. *Journal of American Medical Association,* 1976, *236,* 2643–2644.

Francis, V., Korsch, B. M., & Morris, M. J. Gaps in doctor–patient communication. *New England Journal of Medicine,* 1969, *280,* 535–539.

Kasteler, J., Kane, R. L., Olsen, D. M., & Thetford, C. Issues underlying prevalence of "doctor-shopping" behavior. *Journal of Health and Social Behavior,* 1976, *17,* 328–339.

Commentary

The collection of past-due accounts is a problem faced by most business and professional people. Absence of a clear-cut collection policy produces frequent dilemmas, as demonstrated by the two incidents.

An analysis of the outcome of each incident reveals that the resolution of Mr. A.'s account was negative financially, was anxiety-producing for the physician, staff, and patient, and resulted in a feeling of ill-will between patient and physician. The resolution of Mrs. B.'s account had a positive financial result, had less of an anxiety-producing situation, and resulted in a patient–physician relationship that fostered mutual understanding.

From my experience, I feel that Mr. A.'s account should have been resolved earlier. The episode indicates that this account was of longstanding concern to the physician and his staff and probably the patient. The actions of Mr. A.'s wife added to an already difficult situation. There appeared to be no clear-cut collection policy of past-due accounts adhered to by the physician. To have an account cross one's desk every month presumes the physician is making all the decisions on these types of financial matters. In this instance, the frequency of appearance of this account should have alerted the physician that a problem was imminent, and earlier actions should have been initiated.

Mrs. B.'s account was handled appropriately even though it required using a collector. In both cases, the physician appropriately discussed the problem of the account with the responsible individual before further action was taken.

Problem accounts will always exist for physicians. The most the physician can achieve is minimizing the impact of these past-due accounts on the individuals involved while maintaining the appropriate physician–patient relationships. One way that works effectively is establishing a specific policy on billing and collections that can be implemented by the physician's staff— billing clerk, financial secretary, or office manager. This permits the physician the latitude of becoming involved only in those cases that require a specific decision (send to collection, write off, allow additional time, make personal contact). The physician can then utilize information that he alone may know concerning the patient's particular situation.

The important principle in developing a collection policy is the establishment of a written protocol that is used to resolve overdue accounts. Nothing is gained by merely sending out bills each month with messages that are disregarded by patients. Too often, direct contact with the patient begins with dunning by a collection agency. Early efforts should be more direct to resolve the problem before conflict arises. These include letters and telephone calls by the physician's staff who are specifically assigned this duty. These duties require the time and privacy to do the job well. It should not be an additional duty of the receptionist who tries to fit it in with her other duties.

In family practice, an office should be its own collection agency. If office collection procedures work well, there is little need for outside collection agencies nor does it require a great deal of the physician's time. In those cases where accounts remain unresolved, the physician can then decide whether further action is warranted. If a practice has an effective collection policy that is represented by a collection rate of 90 to 95 percent of all allowable charges, very little will be gained by using outside agencies. Factors that will affect this collection rate include the newness of the practice, location (inner city versus suburban), and the socioeconomic status of the average patient. If your practice is unable to collect the account, in general no one else will be successful.

The discipline of family practice is emphasizing management of a medical practice as a business. Residencies in family practice designate a portion of their curriculum for training in the area of practice management. Most physicians, until very recently, were unfamiliar with many of the business aspects and responsibilities attendant to operating a medical practice. Knowledge of these areas of business, such as personnel, accounting, billing, and collection, permits the management of your practice in a scientific and reasonable manner.

A medical practice that functions efficiently in administrative areas benefits the physician by allowing the physician to control the practice rather than the practice controlling him. It permits additional time for effective, efficient, and high-quality care for one's patients, provides the staff with a quiet, relaxed work setting, and most important, allows the physician to be more in control of his own personal life.

J. David Michaels, B.S., PA-C
Instructor
Medical College of Ohio at Toledo
Toledo, Ohio

Suggested Readings

American Academy of Family Physicians. *Organization and management of family practice*. Kansas City: Author, 1974.

Eisenberg, J. M., & Williams, S. V. *The physician's practice*. New York: John Wiley and Sons, 1980.

33 / Cop Out?

E.R. Triage: Patient Welfare
or Physician Convenience

Background

I have been a family physician for 20 years, 10 of the years practicing in a rural area. I was practicing with an associate in a community of 18,000 people which had no hospital but was seven miles from the center of a large city which had a tertiary university hospital. My associate had the day off and the office was crowded with patients.

The Incident

A teenage boy ran into the office and excitedly told me that his friend, age 16, was lying in a car outside of the office, critically wounded by an accidental firing of a gun which the friend was holding or which was lying on the back seat of the car.

I ran to the car with only my stethoscope, noted that the boy was pale and semiconscious with a rapid pulse, was obviously in pain, and poorly responded to my questioning. The wound was in his abdomen.

I was faced with the decision of taking the boy out of the car into my office where I could start intravenous fluid, bring it to the car and start it there, give him an analgesic injection and/or an injection to raise his blood pressure, or send him immediately to the university hospital.

The emotional impact and strain on me were great. Anything that I would or could do would take five to 10 minutes. I reasoned that the time could best be spent in getting him to the university hospital, a 10- to 15-minute trip. The boy was dead on arrival at the hospital and I had considerable misgivings relative to whether or not I could have done more. I was beginning to feel that rushing him off to the hospital was a "cop out." I had some surgical equipment, experience, oxygen, and facilities for minor surgery available in my office.

Approximately three weeks after the funeral, the father of the deceased boy called and asked, "What kind of doctor are you to ship the boy off to the hospital without treatment, didn't you have any compassion, didn't you want to take time from your busy office, weren't you negligent?"

Discussion

The victim and his family had never been my patients. I had never seen the patient previously so I had no rapport with either patient or family.

It is my feeling that the situation was untenable and that the factor of time was paramount. Had the boys not stopped at the office and had they gone immediately to the university hospital, "stat" surgery may or may not have saved this boy from a traumatic, hemorrhagic death.

How much should one do in a "no win" situation? Does going through the motions of doing something provide legitimacy in terms of satisfying the parents? Does "doing something" assuage the physician's conscience and give him emotional support?

Commentary

This incident illustrates the emotional burden placed on practicing physicians by unrealistic societal expectations regarding the omnipotence of modern medical practice. In this case a physician, practicing alone in an office located 10- to 15-minute's drive from a major university teaching hospital, was called upon to make a rapid medical decision regarding a critically wounded teenager. Although presumably this experienced practitioner had the knowledge and skill to utilize potentially lifesaving diagnostic and therapeutic equipment, he did not have immediate access. Forced to choose between delaying definitive treatment while valuable time was spent in limited therapeutic interventions or sending the patient to the university center without delay, he aptly described the dilemma as a no win situation.

Even retrospectively, not enough information is available to determine the optimal management of this patient. We do not know the exact nature or extent of the boy's injuries. Although we may assume that an abdominal gunshot wound led to significant blood loss, shock, and ultimately exsanguination, we cannot determine the time elapsed between the accident and the presentation at the outlying office. It does seem unlikely that the limited interventions available in the physician's office (primarily minor surgical equipment and injectable analgesics) would have affected the outcome. Many practitioners would advocate starting portable oxygen to be used during transport; some would also advocate attempting to start intravenous fluids during transport. Both of these latter modalities of treatment are employed in many parts of the country by trained Emergency Medical Technicians (Committee on Allied Health, 1977). Regardless of these interventions, it seems unlikely that the boy could have survived.

Two factors are mentioned in the physician's account of the incident that are not directly relevant to the biomedical care of the patient. Both potentially had significant impact on the psychosocial aspects of this case. The first factor is mentioned both by the physician ("the office was crowded with patients") and by the father of the deceased boy ("didn't you want to take time from your busy office?"). Doctors often have a heavy workload. They often find that there is too little time for the "caring" role. In this case the physician could legitimately claim to be busy, but was inappropriately perceived by the relatives of the injured boy as not caring. It seems likely that the pressures of the work setting contributed very little, if at all, to the medical actions taken, but may have contributed a lot to subsequent feelings of guilt on the part of the physician.

The second factor is the lack of previous contact between the physician and the family of the victim. Again, this may not have influenced the medical care that was given, but it had a significant effect on the feelings expressed by the doctor and the family. If the family had been part of the physician's practice, he would probably have been able to serve as a valuable support to the grieving process. Instead, he became the object of displaced anger and frustration from the family of the dead boy. This transfer of blame to the physician, so evident in the increase of malpractice litigation in the past decade, is bolstered by societal views that modern medical practice should be able to guarantee a good result. Although there are certainly many instances when the availability of lifesaving technology may be judged more important than the rapport between patient and care-giver, the quality of the latter must be counted as one factor in the process of medical care delivery. In some ways it is ironic that a family physician, whose practice attempts to provide both technology and caring, should be confronted by an incident where neither type of intervention can be employed.

In the final analysis, there is no clear answer to the no win situation. Based on the probability that hemorrhagic death was inevitable given the nature of the wound and the time lapse between accident and presentation, there was no technological solution to the problem. Had the physician chosen to do something at his office or on the way to the hospital, he might have been able to demonstrate to himself and the family a commitment to providing care even in the face of impossible odds. However, his decision to immediately send the car and its wounded passenger to the hospital is equally defensible from the standpoint of emotional support of a family he never knew. Given the setting in which this incident happened, it seems likely that the physician's conscience may have been tested by accusations of negligence, regardless of the chosen course of action.

It seems important for family practitioners to develop a clear understanding of their limitations as technical providers of medical care and as supportive, caring professionals. Such understanding may come from painful experience, as in this case, or from group discussions of the doctor–patient relationship, such as those advocated by Dr. Michael Balint (1957). Finally, physicians individually and collectively may attempt to educate the public toward a better understanding of these limitations.

David N. Little, M.D.
Assistant Professor of Family Practice
University of Vermont College of Medicine
Burlington, Vermont

References

Balint, M. *The doctor, his patient, and the illness*. New York: International Universities Press, 1957.

The Committee on Allied Health. *Emergency care and transportation of the sick and injured* (2nd ed.). Chicago: American Academy of Orthopaedic Surgeons, 1977.

Commentary

The first question asked by the treating physician in this truly "no win" case is: How much should one do to provide legitimacy in terms of satisfying the family and to assuage his own conscience? Since this is a classic example of a "Catch 22" situation, where no choice will be a winner, it is my feeling that he must do what is morally and ethically correct and, to a certain extent, what he senses will yield the most total good considering all circumstances at the time of the incident. Since this was an ultimate emergency, he only had time for a snap decision based on his knowledge of the health care resources in his community and his long practice background. Doing something to provide legitimacy or to support his conscience does not appear to be a necessary or desirable aspect of the treatment decision in this case, especially under the circumstances described. Doing something might have given him emotional support, but would not likely have changed the outcome in this case.

In regard to the physician's handling of this critical incident, it seems that the majority of physicians would have acted precisely as he did under identical circumstances. However, there are several facts lacking for a complete data base so that one may comment on the judiciousness of his decision: the amount of time between the injury (gunshot wound) to the abdomen and arrival at his office, the availability of paramedical or rescue support in his community and, if available, the time necessary to attain their help, and finally, how the patient was transported to the tertiary care hospital. This physician handled the emergency call immediately by running to the car and noting that the boy was "semiconscious with rapid pulse and pallor, obviously in pain, and poorly responsive to questioning, with an abdominal wound." Rosen (1978, p. 554), in a discussion of hypovolemic shock states,

> It is important to realize that in young, previously healthy victims of trauma there are few recognizable clinical changes until more than 25 percent of the blood volume has been lost. As acute reduction in blood volume continues, the patient's mental state progresses from apathy to coma. As pulmonary changes occur, hypoxia develops with confusion and restlessness and finally, those with greater and more rapid blood loss have a worse prognosis.

Since it is highly likely that this *was* a recent injury, occurring shortly before the patient arrived at the physician's office, the clinical picture presented is one of offering little hope of resuscitation. Our physician had only seconds to decide the correct choice of action and, in my judgment, made the right decision to transport as rapidly as he could to the one place where survival might be possible, a nearby tertiary hospital. The time lag for starting an IV or for bringing the patient into his own office crowded with patients discounts these choices as rational decisions. The only apparent critique would be if support were not given by either the physician or his nurse in personally taking the patient to the hospital in the most expeditious fashion, presuming no immediately adjacent paramedical resource was available. In examining the physician's action by the "retrospectoscope," one may argue that an IV line might have been established in the car in transit and oxygen applied, but in practicality, the possibilities of attaining this are fraught with the difficulties of the motion of the vehicle, the position of the patient, and the likelihood of great difficulty in finding an uncollapsed peripheral vein. Therefore, in summary, it is my strong feeling that the case was handled correctly and as well as a large majority of physicians might have handled it.

The larger issues raised are psychological, ethical, and legal. Psychologically or emotionally, this type of case can be, and apparently was in this instance, devastating to the attending physician. He was presented with a no win situation from the outset and then had his natural feeling of guilt, related to the result of this case, accentuated by the call from the patient's father three weeks later. Obviously, close scrutiny of this case provides one with a near certainty that this was a truly unresolvable, untenable situation without a logical answer and, therefore, no guilt should arise from the logically expected result: the death of the patient before arriving at the hospital. In practicality, it is difficult for a physician to be objective when confronted with this type of incident and not to have the guilt, related to the decision chosen among various options, weigh heavily upon him. Any active physician will have a number of such incidents through his practice lifetime which will have strong impact on him emotionally and, perhaps as well, on his subsequent methods of care. It is obvious that each physician responds differently to emergency situations with an occasional physician attuned to aggressive, decisive action whereas many fine physicians need time for reflection to make judicious decisions even in an emergency. These physicians often have excellent insight into their emergent response and particularly after considerable practice experience find excellent alternatives to handle any emergency. Undoubtedly, if a different course of action had been taken with the same result, a similar or greater amount of guilt would have attended that accident. Furthermore, in the event that this had been a regular patient of this physician and a family with whom he had good rapport, the contacts and subsequent handling of the boy's death would have obviated any kind of family reaction toward the treating M.D. other than their own natural grief. Because there was no rapport here, the father of the victim, quite naturally, shifted some of his anger and perhaps his own guilt for allowing his untrained son to utilize a firearm to the unknown quantity, a physician whose office happened to be on the road of the car bearing his dying son toward help. Finally, an autopsy report is not included in this incident. It is likely that such a report would confirm the hopelessness of the case and help further to assuage the physician's guilt and the father's anger.

It is also important to examine the total situation common in a primary care practice, namely, an extremely busy office with a partner away on vacation or a day off. Some of those other patients were undoubtedly seriously ill, and this fact would have impact on the physician's decision process. It is often quite necessary to quickly shift the responsibility of critical care, particularly in time-consuming incidents, to the best possible resource so that the *most total good* can be performed by the physician. Clearly, this physician's judgment was to shift the responsibility to the tertiary hospital as the best hope after rendering the proper quick assessment.

Ethical issues also assume major significance in this incident. Does the physician have a duty or obligation to treat this new patient at all? Clearly we must consider his obligation to undertake immediate care in measuring his conduct toward the patient and consider all this in the special frame in which the concept of "emergency" draws us. Obviously, the Hippocratic Oath implies such a duty by its statement, "I will follow that system of regimen which, according to my ability and judgment, I consider for the benefit of my patients, and abstain from whatever is deleterious and mischievous." Similarly, the American Medical Association "Principles of Medical Ethics" announce the proposition that "the prime object of the medical profession is to render service to humanity" (AMA, 1971, p. 5). Similarly, "the physician is free to choose whom he will serve. He should, however, respond to any request for his assistance in an emergency or whenever temperate public opinion expects the services" (AMA, 1971, p. 22). Quite obviously, this physician then had an obligation, by good medical ethics, to render emergency aid.

The physician's judgment in this incident also comes under ethical and legal scrutiny. As we have stated, physicians vary in their ability to exercise their best judgment in an emergency, "where one [physician] is confronted with a sudden emergency, without sufficient time to determine with certainty the best course to pursue, he is not held to the same accuracy of judgment as would be required of him as if he had time for deliberation" (*Mississippi Cent R*. v. *Aultman*, 1935). And similarly, "emergency does not lessen the obligation to use care, but merely excuses errors of judgment due to the excitement and necessity for haste produced by the emergency" (*Lachman* v. *Pennsylvania*, 1947). So again, this physician's judgment cannot be faulted on any basis.

Finally, legal considerations are also important in this incident. Considering that the patient in this instance is a minor and the parents are not present, the question arises of consent for treatment. Clearly, by the physician's act of running to the car and assessing the situation, he has rendered treatment regardless of what else is done and has established a contract, even though he has not had any prior relationship with this patient. Factually, this physician is confronted with a true emergency defined by the decision in *Wheeler* v. *Barker* (1949) as "an unforeseen combination of circumstances which call for immediate action." Since this is a true emergency, the physician is, according to Prosser (1964), "privileged to treat under these circumstances because he is reasonably entitled to assume that, if the patient were competent and able to understand the situation, he would consent; thus, it is permissible to act as if consent had been given [and applies to the parents as well]." The Good Samaritan concept may be argued as not applying in this case, since this has been established as a physician–patient contract as noted above. An argument can be made that, in today's medical milieu, defensive medicine is common and this physician might have hesitated to act aggressively fearing malpractice concerns. However, this is easily diffused knowing that as in the case of *Scott* v. *McPheeters* (1939), "the law recognizes that the practice of medicine is not an exact science, that mere mistakes in judgment by a physician do not constitute malpractice." However, as defined in David M. Harney's tome

Medical Malpractice (1973), "the law is designed to compensate those who are victims of treatment falling below the applicable standard of care." As noted above, judgmentally it would appear that this physician has applied a high standard of care in this case.

In summary, it is apparent that in the outlined critical incident, this physician, with his rather broad practical experience, made the most logical and the wisest decision in a truly no win situation. He should have no guilt and should only feel sad that there was not more opportunity to help this unfortunate lad. It is also apparent that similar emergencies arise from time to time in every busy practitioner's life requiring similar emotionally wrenching judgments.

Charles E. Fenlon, M.D.
Associate Professor
Department of Family Medicine and Practice
University of Wisconsin
Appleton, Wisconsin

References

American Medical Association. Principles of medical ethics of the American Medical Association. *Opinion and report of the Judicial Council*. Chicago: Author, 1971

Harney, D. M. *Medical malpractice*. Indianapolis: Allen-Smith Co., 1973.

Lachman v. *Pennsylvania Greyhound Lines*, 160 F 2d 496, 502 (4th Cir., 1947).

Mississippi Cent R. Co v. *Aultman*, 173 Miss. 622, 160 So. 737, 940 (1935).

Prosser, W. L. *Handbook of the law of torts* (4th ed.). St. Paul, Minn.: West Publishing Co., 1964.

Rosen, P. Hypovolemic shock. In G. R. Schwartz, P. Safar, J. H. Stone, P. B. Storey, & D. K. Wagner (Eds.), *Principles and practice of emergency medicine*. Philadelphia: Saunders, 1978.

Scott v. *McPheeters*, 33 Cal. App. 2d 629, 92, P. 2d 678 (1939).

Wheeler v. *Barker*, 92 Cal. App. 2d 776, 785, 208, P. 2d 687 (1949).

34 / Sacrificial Lamb

Medical Malpractice or Legal Manipulation?

Background

For 20 years my practice included obstetrics which I believed, and still believe, is an integral part of family practice. Although time-consuming in the "hurry up and wait" atmosphere of the delivery suite, and often an intrusion into a somewhat structured day, the event of a birth was a most satisfying part of family practice.

I had cared for the T. family for over 12 years with an aggregate of more than 200 visits to the office or home during this period. Mrs. T. was gravida 4 in an unplanned pregnancy which was accepted with reluctance and anxiety. I had delivered two of her last three children, one a difficult footling breech and the other a persistent posterior by forceps rotation. She was almost apologetic but grateful to have these healthy children. She was overweight with the pregnancy, and although not substantiated by blood sugars, she was a potential gestational diabetic. With an otherwise normal prenatal course, vaginal delivery was anticipated.

After a hard labor and slow dilitation, the patient was taken to the delivery room. Examination revealed that the head was descended in a persistent posterior position. Sensing a possible problem, I enlisted the consultative help of the chief of the obstetrical department and his associate, who was also available. The head was rotated with relative ease, but an unpredictable nuchal arm delayed delivery of the baby for several minutes. A large, severely

obtunded female infant was finally delivered with the intentional fracture of
the obstructing arm. After a stormy neonatal course, the baby was discharged
in good condition. The three of us who participated in this most trying
delivery considered the outcome fortuitous under the circumstances.

The Incident
I had always considered the rapport between the T. family and myself
congenial and mutually trustful, but they were upset with the result of this last
delivery and decided to transfer medical care and records to other doctors. In
addition, I never received payment for services rendered. Twelve months
later I was confronted in my waiting room by a court-appointed deputy with a
Summons in Trespass. That same day the announcement of the alleged
malpractice suit was placed in the local papers, a tactic never used before in
my community. The underhanded manner of the attack and the accusations in
the complaint stirred me to anger and incredulity.

I was soon to learn in the painstaking months of legal maneuvering ahead
that, although a malpractice suit may be an affront to the defendant-physician,
it is only a game to be played out by lawyers and judges. What was to me a
challenge to my personal conduct and judgment was to the attorneys a tactical
exercise toward an economic settlement. Any concerted effort to defend me
or to vindicate my course of action was lost to a polite nod.

The case resulted in a settlement only because I was financially not in a
position to throw the decision into the lap of a whimsical jury. I carried low
limits to my malpractice coverage in those early days, and I was not going to
risk exposure to an inordinately large award. The plaintiff received $40,000
shared by my insurance company, the hospital (as co-defendant), and me. I
learned that the expert counsel assigned to me by the carrier had never before
defended in an obstetrical case, and his qualifications as a malpractice lawyer
were moot. My personal attorneys, malpractice specialists, never appeared at
the depositions and were conspiciously absent at the pretrial. For these
services I was billed $9,000, later to be reduced to $6,000 when argued at
arbitration. Although I did not make the decision to deliver the baby vaginal-
ly, I was the only physician named in the suit. My lawyers negligently failed to
name the participating obstetricians in the suit, which constituted legal
malpractice. For this and other pretrial violation of court proceedings I later
sued my own insurance company and their assigned counsel for negligent
conduct. A settlement was reached, without much hassle, for $15,000.

Discussion
The threat of malpractice litigation is a dominant consideration in any doctor–
patient relationship, since awards are made frequently to plaintiffs, whether
capricious or not, without exhaustive proof of negligence. Few doctors can

afford the time or the stomach to fight in a protracted court trial. Insurance carriers, moreover, are quick to settle rather than fight. No matter what, everyone loses this battle, save one—the lawyer.

Through the efforts of some physicians working with the legislature, some minor changes have been made in the system. The crisis, however, far from being over, rears again with the higher premiums, exorbitant awards, and eager attorneys in the wings. As physicians are being asked to increase their coverage limits and catastrophic funds are created to cover the higher awards, the spiral continues. Is the traditional tort system appropriate for medical malpractice? Can insurance companies offer or can physicians afford the astronomical protection into which they are being pressed?

As more and more physicians join the ranks of the sued, there is little consolation left in the axiom that "misery loves company." Perhaps the most devastating effect is that we must practice defensive medicine, a wasteful, redundant, expensive way to practice. Once the doctor experiences the trauma of being sued, he can never again discharge his responsibilities with a relaxed dedication. He becomes suspicious of therapeutic innovations and conservative with declared prognoses. He promises nothing. This has dealt a blow to the optimistic approach and has tempered the consolation of compassion.

Footnote: The unwitting star of this "critical incident," the newborn baby girl, is now a healthy, normal young lady.

Commentary

I would agree with the physician in this case that obstetrics is a delightful and integral part of family practice. The resulting intrusions into the daily routine, while sometimes inopportune, are more often welcome. Indeed the successful delivery of a healthy and wanted baby is one of the most satisfying parts of family practice.

Unfortunately, any practice with a large volume of obstetrical patients is one that will have an occasional high-risk pregnancy and an occasional difficult and complicated delivery. In some instances these are quite predictable, and consultative help may be obtained early in the prepartum course or may be present for the delivery. However, there will always be that small number of cases in which a totally unpredictably difficult delivery will occur. In those cases the physician is not always as fortunate as in this case, where the delivering physician was able to get immediate consultative help from the chief of the obstetrical service and his associate. That was indeed fortuitous, and from the medical standpoint apparently aided in achieving a good medical outcome. It should also have proven to be quite fortuitous from the legal standpoint and should have aided in obtaining a legal outcome favorable to the

attending family physician, who later became the defendant in the malpractice suit.

It has been my experience and one that I have repeatedly observed in
practice and in medicolegal consultations that a good rapport between physician and patient is truly one of the best protections the physician may have
against a malpractice suit. I have personally observed many cases in which the
patient and the patient's family refused to bring suit against a physician whom
they regard as their family physician even if he was clearly liable for some
incident that was legally malpractice.

This case begins with an unplanned pregnancy which was accepted with
reluctance and anxiety by this mother of three small children. Undoubtedly,
this patient had many guilt feelings about this pregnancy, which were reinforced by the difficult labor and stormy neonatal course. These feelings, and
any hostile feelings toward the father, could easily be projected onto the
physician, leading to the desire to punish him, therefore creating a situation
wherein the patient was able to work out her feelings by becoming the plaintiff
and aggrieved party in a lawsuit. Such a person will always be able to find a
lawyer willing to take her case, and this is particularly so if the prospect of high
damages exists.

Based on the facts that are given here, it appears that any damages sustained by the plaintiff, mother or daughter, were not the results of any errors
of omission or commission by the attending physician. Depending on his
experience, it may be that he should have had consultation at an earlier point
in time, but earlier consultation would not have altered the outcome. In the
majority of jurisdictions a less than perfect outcome is not malpractice unless
some negligent action of the attending physician has contributed to that
outcome, nor is it malpractice if the physician errs in judgment so long as the
exercise of that judgment is well-founded in the facts of the case.

It would appear that this incident is one of legal malpractice rather than
medical malpractice because the physician could have been defended on both
medical and legal grounds. This suspicion is strongly reinforced by the fact
that the physician was able to recover $15,000 by suing his own insurance
carrier and that the recovery was by settlement rather than by risking trial.

Commercial carriers are in fact and in their operations totally commercial in
nature. Their approach to the defense of any suit will be predicated upon the
economics of the case. If it is more economical to settle, then that is what the
commercial carrier will usually do. On the other hand, the physician-owned
and -operated insurance carriers are more likely to look at the merits of the
case and to defend against the spurious, unwarranted, or nuisance suit quite
fervently, regardless of the cost, with the apparent intent of discouraging such
frivolous suits. In any circumstances where the defendant physician has
reason to question the competency of counsel provided by a third party, he is
usually well-advised to have his personal attorney present at all times. I am

completely at a loss as to why the personal attorneys described in this case as malpractice specialists were never present at any depositions nor at the pretrial. It would seem that those "personal attorneys" ought to have been sued for legal malpractice, and it is certainly not clear what services they rendered that justified any award.

The birth of a malpractice suit is marked by the delivery of a Summons in Trespass on the named defendants. The drafting of a complaint and the service of a summons should be preceded by an investigation of the factual situation by the plaintiff's attorney. It should include a medical consultation with other physicians in an effort to determine whether the conduct and the judgment exercised by the physician-defendant were indeed deviations from the usual standards of care exercised by other physicians in similar cases. A very important part of the consideration that goes into the initiation of any lawsuit is the amount of damages. The damages are the expected monetary awards either by settlement or by award by the jury. Even in cases of obvious negligence and therefore clear liability, suit will rarely be initiated if the injury to the patient and hence the damages are *de minimis*.

If a patient has been subjected to some action that might be considered malpractice but has not sustained any permanent physical harm or financial loss, then the monetary damages will be small, and it is unlikely that an attorney will pursue the case. However, if the apparent damages are sufficiently high, the plaintiff will easily find some attorney to pursue the action even though the basis of liability may be highly questionable and the possibility of being able to prove that liability is minimal.

It does indeed become a game to be played out by lawyers and judges. It is a game that is played best by those who are not emotionally involved, but who can play with the cool detachment of the professional poker player rather than by one whose moves are dictated by the emotional response to the challenge to his personal conduct and judgment. That emotional response and blindly determined effort to vindicate a given course of action can result in tactical errors that may have adverse effects not anticipated by amateurs to the game.

This amateur defendant quit the game early in order to avoid a jury decision. This decision to quit may have been influenced more by the widespread publicity that large awards receive and remarks by colleagues and others than by an unemotional professional appraisal of possible liability, potential damage, and consideration of what juries are likely to do and, more specifically, of what juries are likely to do in the jurisdiction in which the defendant finds himself.

Juries in rural areas and semirural areas tend to find for the defendant and will do so quite often even in cases where the malpractice is clearly present. On the other hand, in urban areas there is a tendency to find for the plaintiff, even when the medical evidence may not seem to be very convincing. Unlike a criminal case where the burden of proof is to show guilt beyond a reasonable doubt, an action based on allegations of malpractice is a civil action and requires only a preponderance of the evidence to be in favor of the plaintiff in order to permit a finding of liability by the defendant.

The initiation of the suit by a Summons in Trespass is accompanied with the filing of the Complaint or in some jurisdictions the Complaint may be required to be filed shortly thereafter. The Complaint is the legal document that sets forth in detail all of the allegations upon which the plaintiff bases his complaint. This document will set forth the claims of the plaintiff in language that is very offensive to the physician-defendant and which would often be libelous if the words were taken at face value or uttered in some other situation. These words, read in the legal context, generally have a somewhat different meaning than that which is ordinarily given to them. Likewise, the claims for damages will invariably describe the alleged injury to the plaintiff in such terms that any lay person who reads the Complaint would wonder that the plaintiff ever survived, and having survived, how the plaintiff managed to deal with the terrible pain, horrible suffering, and grievous mental anguish as alleged in his complaint. In the vast majority of complaints the approbation of the physician-defendant is quite real and often the initial emotional response that is evoked is sufficiently long lasting so as to preclude the physician from ever becoming a truly good witness in his own defense.

There is another aspect of the games that lawyers and judges play that is poorly understood by the physician population, and it is one which leads to a great deal of frustration and often evokes an angry response when it is understood. It is that neither truths nor facts as they are perceived by either plaintiff or defendant are recognized truths or facts in the course of the trial of a case unless they can be brought before the finder of facts, whether it be a judge or a jury, in a manner that falls within the rules of evidence in the jurisdiction in which the case is being tried. Often that which is perceived by the physician-defendant as being a true statement and a fact may not necessarily enter into the deliberations leading to the final outcome if that fact cannot be brought before the judge or the jury in the proper manner. It often appears that a trial is not so much a search for truth as it is a contest to influence the outcome by virtue of those facts which may be brought forth by either party while making every effort to limit the opponent's presentation of those facts of the case which would be favorable to his client. It is certainly not a game to be played by amateurs, particularly by those who are so directly involved as to become overly emotional about any one of the multitude of little battles and scrimmages that are only a part of the overall trial.

This case is an illustration of legal malpractice. The physician-defendant was able to recover a substantial sum of money based on the same principles that apply in questions of medical malpractice. There was legal negligence on the part of the attorney and that negligence is founded in his departure from the usual standards of care in the handling of such cases. In this incident, quite clearly the chief of service and his associate should have been brought into the defense of the family physician. This could have been done by having them appear either as expert witnesses or as additional defendants. The failure to name those potential additional defendants in the original suit may have been a tactical matter, a part of the gamesmanship of the plaintiff's attorney, but based on the facts of the case given here, their presence was quite essential to an adequate defense.

I have for many years held the view that the counsels for the defendants in malpractice actions are really counsels for the insurance carriers and only secondarily for defendants. Many or perhaps even most defense attorneys that I have had the opportunity to observe in action do in fact perform creditably well and truly exert their best efforts for the defendant. There have been those instances in which the defense was not all that it could have been and in which the defense attorney was not putting forth the best defense available for his client.

One of the reasons for carrying malpractice insurance has always been in part to assure the presence of a defense attorney with expertise in malpractice law and to insure against the financial burden created by the cost of defending an action in malpractice. It is still advisable in the event of a malpractice suit that a physician have his own personal attorney present or available to review procedures at every step of the way. Alternately, one may submit one's fate to the mercy of the attorney selected by the insurance carrier, and thereafter to carefully observe, note, and record all the actions of that individual and in the event that the outcome is unfavorable or not as promised, then to engage in what has become the great American pastime of litigation. Physicians too can ask for second opinions and can second-guess the legal experts, and if it seems that there is a deviation from the standards for defense of a medical malpractice and if the physician is found liable as a result, then a suit for legal malpractice is in order.

Roland T. Keddie, M.F., J.D.
Chairman
Department of Emergency Services
McKeesport Hospital
McKeesport, Pennsylvania

Commentary

It is truly a harrowing and unpleasant experience to be sued for money damages for something you allegedly did wrong. Whether the allegations of wrongdoing are meritorious or not, the person sued is usually thrust into an unfamiliar world of liability insurance, lawyers, judges, and the adversary system of justice.

This experience is especially traumatic and distasteful for a physician who is sued for medical malpractice. By definition, a medical malpractice lawsuit is filed by a patient (or more likely a former patient) with whom the physician has had personal contact in a effort to help, and often with whom the physician has had a close, longstanding personal relationship. This factor, which is frequently absent in other types of civil cases, tends to cause a unique, long-lasting, emotional reaction such as expressed by this doctor: "This [medical malpractice experience] has dealt a blow to an optimistic approach and has tempered the consolation of compassion."

Furthermore, a malpractice suit is commonly viewed by the physician as an indictment of his competence and as a substantial threat to his professional reputation which he has worked so hard to establish. As a result, the sued physician usually seeks vindication and, sometimes, revenge.

Additional factors which often contribute to a sued physician's anxiety and anger are (1) his unfamiliarity with the liability insurance system, (2) his unfamiliarity with the adversary system for resolving civil disputes, and (3) his gut feeling that it is just plain unfair for him to be sued when he has done his best under difficult circumstances. After all, a good result can never be guaranteed in medicine.

Recognition and consideration of these understandable anxiety- and anger-producing factors may help a physician to better cope with a malpractice lawsuit when one is filed. Initially, it is important for the physician to understand that, like it or not, some system of recovery for injuries caused by medical malpractice is here to stay and that the chance of being sued at least once in one's career is considerable. Simply a realization and awareness of this prospect will not only assist the physician in dealing with a lawsuit but will go a long way toward reducing the chance of being sued. Despite the doctor's observation that "there is little consolation left in the axiom that 'misery loves company,' " the sued physician should remember that no doctor, however eminent, competent, and careful, is immune from (and few will be spared from) the sword of malpractice litigation.

It is, therefore, essential that a physician obtain the best professional liability insurance coverage affordable if he is to be protected from the very real threat of personal and professional financial disaster. This brings us to the question raised in this incident: "Can insurance companies offer or can physicians afford the astronomical protection into which they are being pressed?" This writer believes the current answer is yes. Good malpractice insurance is now readily available at generally affordable premiums.

The medical malpractice crisis of the mid-1970s arose out of a large and rather sudden increase in malpractice lawsuits and awards, coupled with huge liability premium increases. Some doctors even experienced an inability to obtain any coverage because several insurance companies, in a panic, stopped writing medical malpractice coverage. Although the number of malpractice lawsuits and the size of awards have continued to increase, the insurance side of the crisis has seemingly subsided due to a better understanding and handling of the situation by insurers. For example, a medical malpractice insurance association set up by the Ohio Legislature in 1975 to assure the availability of affordable and adequate coverage to Ohio physicians is in the process of dismantlement because private malpractice insurance companies are now so numerous and competitive.

As to affordability of good coverage, physicians are forced to pass the expense of malpractice premiums on to their patients in the form of higher fees. They simply cannot afford to be "caught," as the doctor in this incident was, without adequate professional liability coverage.

The doctor in this incident carried low liability limits. Insufficient coverage not only exposed him to the risk of personal financial loss but placed added pressure on him and his carrier to settle the lawsuit to avoid that risk. This situation can lead to an unreasonably high settlement payment and may even deprive the doctor of an opportunity to present a good defense. Therefore, it is imperative to secure and maintain all the coverage that is realistically needed. Don't wait to be sued, as the doctor in this incident did, to find out whether your coverage is (in)adequate. A periodic check with your malpractice insurance agent should eliminate the problem of being underinsured.

This doctor was also forced personally to contribute to a multi-party settlement of only $40,000 and incurred personal attorney's fees of $9,000 (reduced to $6,000 at fee arbitration). This was probably because he had a deductible or retention policy. Such a policy not only requires an up-front contribution by the physician but it frequently requires the involvement of the physician's personal attorney, at the physician's own expense, especially if the amount of the deductible or retention is substantial. Although the premium may be a little higher, a nondeductible policy which provides full coverage up to the policy limit will generally preclude these problems.

The doctor in this incident is also concerned about the inability to defend because insurance carriers are quick to settle, rather than fight." Keep in mind that it is the insurance company's money that is usually at stake. For obvious reasons, insurance companies do not approve or pay settlements without careful evaluation of the risk, loss exposure, and expense of formal resolution by trial or arbitration. For those physicians who are, nevertheless, particularly concerned about being "sold out," there are still policies available which give the physician the right to veto settlement proposals.

Another question raised in this incident is whether the traditional tort system is appropriate for medical malpractice. Under traditional tort law a person is generally liable if he fails to exercise ordinary care under the circumstances and his failure to do so proximately causes injury or death. This fundamental concept is designed both to compensate those injured by another's negligence and to make individuals responsible and accountable for their acts.

Medical malpractice is simply a term which encompasses the professional negligence of a physician, hospital, or other medical practitioner. Traditionally, it has been treated as just another type of negligence action. Few physicians would disagree with the basic tort principle that a physician, like all individuals and professionals, including lawyers, should be responsible and accountable for injuries and damages caused by his negligence or lack of due care. (The doctor in this incident should not be critical of this principle as he brought a successful legal malpractice action against his lawyers for their professional negligence.) There is, however, sharp disagreement on what is medical "negligence" or "malpractice" and what the ground rules should be to determine whether or not a doctor is liable.

In the midst of the medical malpractice crisis, state legislatures, under pressure from doctors, hospitals, insurance companies, and the public, were forced to deal with these questions. At issue was the patient's right to seek and obtain compensation for injuries negligently inflicted by physicians versus the public interest in assuring the availability and delivery of adequate medical care and services.

Most legislatures acknowledged the uniqueness of medical malpractice litigation and sought to modify existing procedures for bringing and pursuing malpractice claims. As a result, many states have created, by statute, a separate and distinct cause of action for medical malpractice, with a new set of rules, standards, and procedures designed to eliminate many of the problems encountered in the traditional tort system. These enactments commonly shorten the statute of limitations, set forth stricter pleading requirements, provide for mandatory arbitration, set forth expert witness qualifications, and limit the amount of damages recoverable for pain and suffering, to mention but a few of the changes. Although the basic principles of tort law still apply, such legislative changes can hardly be called "minor."

It is still too early to determine whether these changes will work as intended. However, it is this writer's opinion that a modified tort system, based upon fault (negligence), is the appropriate way to handle medical malpractice claims.

In conclusion, the sword of a medical malpractice lawsuit is, indeed, sharp. However, proper preparation for its thrust will help soften the blow and, hopefully, will prevent the experience from taking the edge off the physician's optimism, compassion, and relaxed dedication.

Timothy D. Krugh, J.D.
Associate Attorney
Robinson, Curphey, and O'Connell
Toledo, Ohio

Index